Brain Food

Recipes for Success in School, Sports, and Life

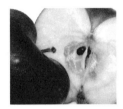 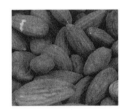 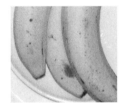

VICKI GUERCIA CARUANA and KELLY GUERCIA HAMMER

M. Evans

Lanham · New York · Boulder · Toronto · Plymouth, UK

Published by M. Evans
An imprint of The Rowman & Littlefield Publishing Group, Inc.
4501 Forbes Boulevard, Suite 200, Lanham, Maryland 20706

Estover Road
Plymouth PL6 7PY
United Kingdom

Distributed by NATIONAL BOOK NETWORK

Library of Congress Cataloging-in-Publication Data

Caruana, Vicki.
    Brain food : recipes for success in school, sports, and life / Vicki Guercia Caruana
and Kelly Guercia Hammer. — 1st m. evans ed.
        p. cm.
    ISBN-13: 978-1-59077-100-6 (pbk. : alk. paper)
    ISBN-10: 1-59077-100-1 (pbk. : alk. paper)
        1. Children—Nutrition. 2. School children—Food. 3. Diet therapy for children.
    4. Cookery. I. Hammer, Kelly Guercia, 1970-. II. Title.
    RJ206.C37 2007
    641.5'622—dc22   2007002754

⑩™ The paper used in this publication meets the minimum requirements of American
National Standard for Information Sciences—Permanence of Paper for Printed Library
Materials, ANSI/NISO Z39.48-1992.

Manufactured in the United States of America.

To my grandmother, Rose Guercia,
who taught me that food is more than sustenance—
it's family. (V.G.C.)

To my parents, Charles and Eileen Guercia,
who believed and taught me the importance
of living "everything in moderation." (K.G.H.)

contents

PART I   MIND–BODY CONNECTIONS

PART II   GROWING BODIES/GROWING MINDS

PART III   recipes for success

Chapter 10. Lunch: The Lunch Bunch 130

Chapter 11. Dinner: Dinner Delights 142

Chapter 12. Snacks: Morning Glories and Brain Breaks 153

Foreword

Have you ever noticed that when you eat a balanced, healthy meal that instead of feeling lethargic or out of it, you feel much more alert and ready to go? Some would say that we eat to fuel our bodies—this includes our brains. Fueling the brain *properly* with the *right* nutrients can make the difference between achieving optimal brain development or mental impairment.

Mom always told us to eat breakfast. More than likely she told you that breakfast is the most important meal of the day. Not only can breakfast be delicious, but it can help a child obtain better scores on his or her school tests (compared with those who skip breakfast) and improve overall cognitive development. There is no great secret ingredient to *Brain Food*, just great knowledge, intimate experience, clinical research, and the applied practice of what this book teaches with our own children.

To understand how to eat nutrient-dense foods that are lower in overall calories, reduced in free sugars and salt is a great gift we as parents should share with our children. These days it's up to parents to take responsibility to teach children how to eat for optimal health, performance, and enjoyment rather than let television or the Internet influence the daily menu. Children follow and mimic what they see done from people they consider mentors (even if they don't admit it). Thus, how you eat, what kind of exercise you do, even the types of clothes you wear will have and make an impression on your children and those around you. Lead by example! It's a great way to be the best teacher for your children.

DOUGLAS S. KALMAN, Ph.D., RDM FACN
Director Nutrition
Miami Research Associates
Adjunct Professor
New York Chiropractic College

acknowledgments

WITHOUT THE FOLLOWING people in my life, this book would not be in your hands. Our mother was a huge part of the inception of this idea. Having worked as a school lunch lady for seventeen years, she shared with me the inside scoop about what goes on in schools at lunchtime. It benefited me as a teacher and later as a parent sending my children off to school. Her insights were the driving force behind this book, and I'm glad she knew it was going to be a reality before she passed away. I would also like to thank my sister and coauthor, Kelly Hammer, whose expertise and well-balanced approach to family nutrition opened my eyes to truths about nutrition that remained hidden to me until she shed light on them. Her philosophies that everything should be done in moderation and that nutrition should be customized to the needs of the consumer are the obvious underpinnings of this book. Finally, I would like to acknowledge the wholehearted support and insights of our editor, P. J. Dempsey, at M. Evans and Company who ran with this idea in both a professional and enthusiastic manner. (V.C.)

I would like to acknowledge and thank my husband, Stanley, and my children, Jacob and Abigail, for their constant love and support throughout the making of this book. Also, a big thank you goes to Leigh Ayling, a dear friend of mine and a "second mom" to my children during the past year. Without my sister, Vicki Caruana, this book would have never become a reality. Her insight into the needs of children from the perspective of a teacher and mother is what brought to life the concept of *Brain Food*. To everyone at M. Evans and Company, particularly P. J. Dempsey, our editor, thank you for all your hard work and creativity in making *Brain Food* a success. (K.H.)

INTRODUCTION

Balance. It's all about living a well-balanced life. Society tosses and turns us from one extreme to the other, when all we really need to live successful, productive, healthy, and happy lives is moderation. As parents we are always on the hunt for something that can give our children an edge in life. At the same time we are on a desperate search for simplicity and harmony in our homes. So much of what our children encounter and experience seems completely out of our control, so if there is something we can control, we should. What and how our children eat is very much within our control. We're the ones who buy the food, after all! When we eat right, we are more likely to feel right and do right.

There is a direct connection between what we eat and how well we learn. We already know the effect some foods have on our children's behavior, but the effect they have on their ability to learn is not as commonly understood. So many children struggle to get all they can out of their educational experiences, and there are contributing factors to that difficulty. When ruling out possible culprits, it's important to equally consider their diets. From before birth, brain development is dependent on nutritional intake. A fetus will generally take what he needs from his mother's body in the form of nutrients, even if that means depleting her reserves. But once a child is born, healthy eating is not automatic. Parents must intentionally supply what growing children need to develop both physically and mentally.

With a little bit of understanding and a lot of practice, feeding your child right becomes "doable" and is no longer a daunting task. The information in this book is a result of the combined efforts of a family nutritionist and an educator. Your nutritionist, Kelly Hammer, has worked with many different families with a wide range of nutritional needs, from curing the sugar-addicted kid to addressing the "diabetic's dilemma." Through her years of nutritional consulting and research, teaching school, and raising her own children, Kelly has seen firsthand the importance of a well-balanced lifestyle, which includes optimal nutrition and exercise. Your educator, Vicki Caruana, has spent much of her career both in and outside the classroom working with parents to set their children up for success. The nutrition–brain connection is well documented and an integral part of learning. Vicki helps you make those all-important connections for yourself so that you can set your child up to succeed.

It is our hope and intention in this book to both equip and empower parents to embrace their role as "nutrition managers" by providing the science behind the concepts of nutrition and learning, the relevant ties to daily life, and the tools to feed their families well. This book is a valuable resource that you will turn to again and again like a trusted friend for information and support. We can't rely on other people to feed our children the way they need to be fed. We can't close our eyes to the fact that many of our children lead sedentary yet stressful lives. We can help change that—just by choosing to feed them according to their needs. Eating is a family affair. That's why we thought it appropriate that two sisters, who know what your life is like, could help you decipher this recipe for success.

Remember: everything in moderation. This book is for the long haul, not the quick fix. It will be your new best friend, providing simple, steadfast wisdom to carry you through the challenges you face to feed your child right in these fast-food times. You can do it right. You can do it now.

Bon appétit!

PART I

mind–body
connections

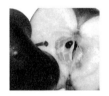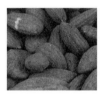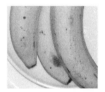

Chapter 1

FEED THE BODY AND THE MIND

Tastes are made, not born.

MARK TWAIN

Laurie downed her second cup of coffee by the time her three kids stumbled out of their bedrooms and into the kitchen. Her oldest, Jeremy, stood motionless in front of the open refrigerator.

"What's there to eat?" he said.

"Just have some cereal," Laurie said while tying the shoes of 6-year-old Stephanie, who carefully munched her fruit cereal bar.

"But I'm hungry. Cereal isn't enough," Jeremy complained.

"We don't have time for this right now, Jeremy," she said. "Just pick something."

"There's nothing good. I don't like that shredded wheat stuff," he said.

Laurie lifted 15-month-old Lizzie out of the high chair, wiped her face, pulled on her jacket, and sat her on the couch. Stephanie sucked her second juice box dry and asked for more.

"No, that's enough, Steph," Laurie said. "Go brush your teeth. It's time to go to school."

"What about eggs, Mom? Can you make me a couple of eggs?" Jeremy asked.

"We only have 10 minutes before we're out the door, Jeremy. Just grab a fruit bar and then go brush your teeth," Laurie said while pouring her third cup of coffee into her travel mug.

Jeremy let out a sigh that could have knocked over a skyscraper. "Whatever," he said and went to brush his teeth.

Before getting out of the car at school, Jeremy pulled a piece of paper folded into a tiny square. "Here. I forgot to give this to you yesterday. It's from Mrs. Little."

Laurie sat in the car and read the note his teacher wrote. It was just like all the others.

Dear Mrs. Taylor,

Jeremy is a joy to have in my class but has trouble focusing on the task at hand and has to be reminded multiple times to get to work. He seems especially tired in the mornings. Is there a way you can make sure he gets to bed a little earlier?

Sincerely,
Meg Little

What is she talking about? Jeremy goes to bed at 8:30 P.M. every night. He gets plenty of sleep. What could be wrong that he can't focus? Laurie looked at her watch. She had 2 hours before Lizzie's nap time.

"I'll just run errands," she said out loud to herself. "I have no energy to go to the gym anyway."

STAMP OF APPROVAL

It's too bad that there are no quality control inspectors who come into our homes and give us that stamp of approval. Maybe it's a good thing since most of us are doing just the bare minimum to get by. We're tired, way too busy, and basically ignorant about what it takes to feed our children right. If someone came into our homes to see what we stocked in our pantries and refrigerators, most likely they'd throw us off the assembly line and into the reject bin.

The hype bombarding us every day about childhood obesity, epidemic onset of diabetes, attention deficit/hyperactivity disorder (ADHD), and a wide variety of eating disorders should scare us into nutritional compliance. But instead it seems to have desensitized us to the fact that we're not doing a very good job at feeding our children. And that's no surprise since as grown-ups we're not eating very well, either. Some of us skip breakfast and would prefer to live off of an intravenous drip of caffeine (guilty here!). Some of us still haven't met a vegetable we like. Some try out diet after diet as if they're speed dating—we give it a week, and if it doesn't work, we move on to something else. Some of us are already paying for our food choices. We're tired all the time. We have difficulty focusing on tasks at work or at home. We're not sleeping well. Our legs twitch in the middle of the night, and we don't recover from illness very quickly. Not to mention the early onsets of diabetes, heart disease, and a host of other diseases. And our children eat just like us.

set them up to succeed

We would like to challenge you to consider one other life-altering fact before you throw up your hands in resignation and say, "What's a mother to do?" When you feed your child's body, you're also feeding his mind. Basically, you're feeding him his future one bite at a time. Many educators can tell who eats breakfast and who doesn't. They suspect who had a protein-rich, stick-to-your-bones type of breakfast and who had air-puffed sugar-and-food-coloring corn balls. How do they know? Children who sleep in class, are lethargic, have difficulty staying on task, are irritable or otherwise bouncing off the classroom walls are the obvious cases. But there are those whose telltale signs are more subtle. Mood swings, poor participation in outside activities, low stamina, indecision, and even mild depression can be results of poor nutrition.

Right now our children's success is measured by how well they learn. School is their job. Parents all over the planet want the best for their children. We want to give them a leg up, help them get a step ahead, set them up to succeed. There are so many things about their learning and school situations that we just can't control, but food choices are very much within our control. Take the reins now and plan a recipe for success for your children that feeds their mind as it feeds their body.

can you do one without the other?

The fact is that when you feed your body you *are* feeding your brain. Since the brain is an organ, it receives the same nutrients that the rest of the body receives when we eat. Feeding and nourishing are two different activities. In order to *nourish* something, you have to find out what it needs in order to function properly and at optimal capacity and then be quite intentional about providing for those needs. Feeding is just the scooping of foodstuffs into a body like coal is shoveled into the gaping hole of a furnace.

We talk about *heart*-healthy diets containing little cholesterol and fats to promote blood circulation and protein to build heart muscle, both of which contribute to a healthy heart that pumps up your life. Unfortunately, we usually don't pay attention to a heart-healthy diet until it screams for attention when diagnosed with heart disease. As always, we then have a choice of whether to follow dietary guidelines or not, but at least we no longer walk around ignorant. The American Heart Association's recommendations promote nutrition and exercise guidelines that together offer a preventative cure and a chance at living a long, healthy life—success!

IF THE BRAIN AIN'T HAPPY, AIN'T NO BODY HAPPY

Brain-healthy diets actually give you a more concentrated dose of success. The complex workings of a human life are coordinated by the most important organ in the body—the brain. Brain-healthy diets include carbohydrates that power the brain's functions, proteins that provide good mental health and balance, certain fats that protect the brain and make it easier for the brain to communicate with the rest of the body, certain vitamins and minerals that promote memory and communication, and water that increases alertness and concentration. You've heard the saying "If Mama ain't happy, ain't nobody happy." Consider this: if the brain ain't healthy, ain't no body healthy.

We can't see our brains, so it's difficult to tell how and when they need to be cared for. Brains must function properly if the rest of the body is to function. If we starve our bodies, we starve our minds. Our decision making becomes impaired and our reactions sluggish. If we want our children to succeed—at school, in relationships with others, for life—then we need to set them up for success by feeding them right.

NATURE OR NURTURE: DO KIDS EAT RIGHT NATURALLY, OR DO THEY GRAVITATE TO WHAT IS BAD FOR THEM?

"She'd eat chips all day if I let her."

"If my son had his way, he'd eat dessert all day every day."

"If I didn't stay on her, she wouldn't eat at all."

Kids may not always make the best choices when on their own, but one thing is for sure: they will eat when they're hungry. Survival demands it. They will eat, but what they eat and how much they eat is up to you when they are with you.

Naturally all babies start consuming carbs (complex sugars) even before they're born. When exactly does nurture take its role? Almost immediately. Even if your child has a birth defect or some kind of disability, you have the choice to make the best of the situation now and improve her quality of life for the future. A child with Down syndrome can be a child with Down syndrome high on sugar (which exacerbates erratic behavior) or a child with Down syndrome who eats nutritious foods that increase her abilities.

Parents have the power when it comes to providing healthy food choices for children. Sometimes it seems like children have a natural tendency toward sugar-soaked snacks, but it's only because that's what's available to them. Consider a time in history when people only ate what they harvested or raised on the farm. This doesn't mean people didn't have a sweet tooth; it means that they ate what was around. Even farmers wrestled with kids who ate too much bread, drank the cream instead of the milk, or wouldn't touch their Brussels sprouts (no offense to those who love them). The control we have as parents is powerful. Provide healthy choices, offer them variety, make it appealing (especially if it's new to them), and you increase the chances that they will eat healthy food. If one vegetable isn't accepted, try another. And remember that tastes change over time. Just because they reject broccoli now doesn't mean they'll reject it in a couple of years. As parents, we can provide opportunities for healthy eating even if no one else does. You may not be pleased with the school lunch offerings or what your son ate at his friend's house or the fact that Grandma always takes them out for fast food. Those things are out of your control. But what they eat within our homes is very much within our control.

Show Me the Freshness

Become accustomed to looking for and reading the "use by" date on packages, especially on perishables, such as salad makings, meat, poultry, and dairy products. Check "on sale" items carefully.

WHAT YOU SEE IS WHAT YOU EAT

Basically we all eat what is available to us. Look in your pantry and refrigerator right now, and you will see what you've made available to yourself and your family to eat. Vicki admits that her snack of choice is more often than not chocolate. "I crave the endorphin rush chocolate provides (and I can stop whenever I want, really)." But she also knows if she eats chocolate every time she wants it, she will suffer in other ways: "I'll experience a sugar crash and brain drain shortly thereafter, my tummy doesn't process the rest of my food very smoothly for the rest of the day, and my eyes will get puffy." Kids experience similar consequences for not eating right, and most likely they will happen right in the middle of the school day. Brain drain is bad enough, but brain drain in the middle of math class can be catastrophic.

NUTRITION AND LEARNING: DOES IT REALLY MAKE A DIFFERENCE?

Educators have known for almost 100 years the link between nutrition and learning. Hot lunches (and now breakfast) at school hasn't been included during the school day for the convenience of parents. Education proponents realized that many children came to school hungry and were then unable to concentrate on their schoolwork. They provided a hot, nutritious lunch so that students were better equipped to learn. Trying to teach children all they have to learn without proper nutrition is like trying to train a horse to jump a hurdle with only three legs: it's a definite handicap.

Since the brain orchestrates the functions of the rest of the body, it stands to reason that if it is hindered from doing its job, we become hindered from doing ours. Brain-based learning advocates offer many educators and parents a way to increase the brain's potential to learn and retain information. But just as a high-performance car is equipped with options to make it run faster, smoother, and longer, our brains can't perform at optimum levels without the right fuel. Both will sputter, stall, or overheat before reaching their goals.

THE MORE YOU KNOW

Schools are paying attention to the research. Water bottles are now accepted accessories, nutritious snacks are offered on state testing days, and children are encouraged to partake in the breakfast program. Teachers want your children to succeed just as much as you do. They're doing what they can do; now we need to do the rest. We can limit their sugar, salt, and cholesterol intake because these things block the brain's ability to absorb much-needed vitamins and minerals. We can increase their water intake and offer water-packed fruits and vegetables that help the brain absorb vital nutrients. We can limit or even eliminate caffeine from our children's diets since it disrupts brain messages sent to the rest of the body. We can accept the truth that what they eat affects how well they learn and purchase food that reflects that truth.

Low-Fat Desserts

The manufacturer often compensates for the fat by adding more sugar. "Low-fat" is not the same as "low-calorie."

FOOD CHOICES: THE GOOD, THE BAD, AND THE UGLY

Knowing why you should provide a brain-healthy diet is one thing. Knowing *what* to buy is quite another. You don't have to become a nutritionist or dietitian to find out what's good for your body and brain and what isn't. The *best* foods include the highest nutrient content possible in them (you get more bang for your buck or mouthful). The *worst* foods are high in sugar, salt, and cholesterol and inhibit the absorption of good nutrients. (For a detailed list of foods that may cause hyperactivity or slow learning in children, see appendix D, Nutritional Tables and Charts.) Consider the following lists the next time you go shopping.

THE BEST

MEATS

Roast beef (round)	Flank steak	Porterhouse
Lamb (leanest cut)	Pork (leanest cut)	Veal (leanest cut)
Chicken (light or dark meat)	Quail	Pheasant
Filet mignon	London broil	Sirloin steak
Loin chops	Fresh ham	Shoulder chops
Cornish hen	Turkey (young, light or dark meat)	T-bone steak
		Venison

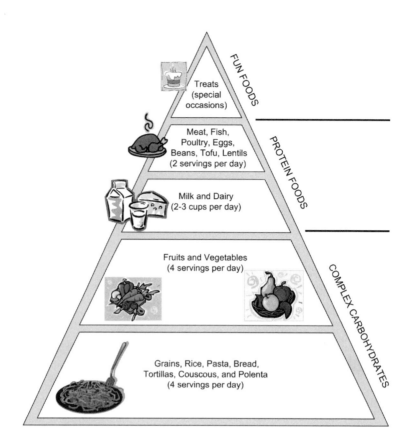

FUN FOODS

Treats
(special
occasions)

PROTEIN FOODS

Meat, Fish,
Poultry, Eggs,
Beans, Tofu, Lentils
(2 servings per day)

Milk and Dairy
(2-3 cups per day)

Fruits and Vegetables
(4 servings per day)

COMPLEX CARBOHYDRATES

Grains, Rice, Pasta, Bread,
Tortillas, Couscous, and Polenta
(4 servings per day)

DAIRY

Buttermilk	Cottage cheese	Ricotta
Yogurt, plain	Farmer cheese	Whole milk
Pot cheese	Skim milk	Parmesan cheese
Dry milk	Mozzarella cheese	

GRAINS

Arrowroot flour	Spaghetti	Macaroni
Pasta (Neapolitan style)	Unbleached flour	Rye flour
Stone-ground whole wheat flour	Cornstarch	Whole wheat pastry flour
Buckwheat flour	Linguini	
	Dry yeast	

LEGUMES/NUTS

Dried beans	Lentils	Nut butters
Almonds	Walnuts	Sunflower seeds
Dried peas	Sesame seeds	Tofu
Peanuts		

FRUITS

Apples	Cherries	Grapes
Mangos	Nectarines	Oranges
Apricots	Cantaloupe	Grapefruit
Peaches	Raisins	Papaya
Bananas	Cranberries	Guava
Pears	Raspberries	Honeydew melon
Black cherries	Dates	Pineapple
Plums	Limes	Juices (fresh)
Blueberries	Figs	Strawberries
Prunes	Lemons	

VEGETABLES

Artichoke	Okra	Sweet potatoes
Bamboo shoots	Cabbage	Parsnips
Asparagus	Sprouts	Tomatoes
Dark leafy lettuce	Cauliflower	Peas
Broccoli	Pumpkin	Tomato Juice
Escarole	Celery	Pea pods
Beets	Radishes	Vegetable juices
Green beans	Corn	Potatoes
Carrots	Squash (summer/winter)	Zucchini
Eggplant		Rhubarb
Cucumber	Green peppers	Yams

FATS

Butter (sweet, no salt)	Cottonseed oil	Virgin olive oil
Corn oil	Sesame oil	Safflower oil
Soybean oil	Peanut oil	Walnut oil

CONDIMENTS/SPICES

Allspice	Nutmeg	Poppy seeds
Ginger	Watercress	Cumin
Tarragon	Bay leaves	Rosemary
Aniseed	Onion	Dill
Marjoram	Wine vinegar	Sage
Thyme	Cardamom seeds	Fennel seeds
Balsamic vinegar	Oregano	Shallots
Mustard seeds	Cayenne	Garlic
Vanilla bean	Parsley	Smoked yeast
Basil	Chives	

THE WORST

BAKED GOODS

Bagels	Baking soda	Cakes
Cookies	Croissants	Pastries
Pumpernickel	Rye bread	White bread
Baking powder	Brownies	Crackers
Corn bread	Doughnuts	Pies
Rolls	Sweet rolls	

BEVERAGES

Alcoholic beverages	Diet drinks	Soft drinks, including cola drinks
Cocoa	Instant drinks	
Coffee		Tea

CONDIMENTS, SAUCES, DRESSINGS

Chili sauce	Steak sauce	Ketchup
Soy sauce	Horseradish	Mayonnaise
Chutney	Tabasco sauce	Prepared mustards

DESSERTS

Candy	Custards	Ice cream
Jellies	Mousses	Sherbets
Chocolate	Flavored gelatin	Ices
Jams	Puddings	Syrups

FATS AND OILS

Artificially colored butter	Hardened white vegetable shortening	Lard
Coconut oil	Margarine with additives	Palm oils

DAIRY

Coffee creamers	High-fat cheeses (e.g., Brie, Muenster, and Gorgonzola)	Processed cheeses
Whipped cream		Flavored yogurts

MEATS AND POULTRY

Bacon	Fatty cuts of meat	Sausages
Capon	Goose	Self-basting poultry
Duck	Ham	

FISH

Caviar	Fish sticks	Smoked fish (including salmon, Nova Scotia salmon, finnan haddie)

PRODUCE

Almonds*	Corn*	Spinach*
Avocados	Kale*	Turnips*
Beets*	Mustard greens	Watercress*
Cabbage	Rutabaga*	

(*Items consumed raw may inhibit certain vitamin and mineral absorption.)

All canned, instant, and prepared foods, mixes, and stuffing contain additives that can inhibit the optimal function of your child's brain and body.

GROWING BODIES, GROWING MINDS

Children's bodies grow little by little, and so do their minds. It's actually amazing how much they learn in such a short period of time.

Within the first 3 years of life, they learn how to walk, talk, play, and interact with their surroundings. During the early weeks and months of gestation, mothers are encouraged to eat certain foods and avoid others in order to promote optimum brain development in their child. We stop smoking, decrease or completely cut out caffeine, drink more milk, eat more protein, and avoid medications, drugs, and alcohol and exposure to chemicals and pesticides. Why? Because it can increase the likelihood of brain damage or delayed development. Once a child is born, his need for proper nutrition continues as he develops mentally and physically.

Each age and stage in a child's development includes specific milestones and situations. Each requires at least an elementary awareness of nutritional needs in order to facilitate children's growth intellectually, physically, and socially. We had complete control over their food intake when they were in the womb. We can still have a great deal of influence as they continue to live and grow in the outside world. The habits we help them develop now will hopefully follow them into adulthood and the raising and feeding of their own children. And if they develop special concerns during this life journey, we can be prepared to deal with those, too.

The chapters to follow offer a great deal of insight into the physical, nutritional, and learning needs of children from birth to 18.

Weigh Your Bread

In general, the heavier the bread, the more nutrients it contains. When in the bread aisle at your local supermarket, compare breads by holding a loaf in each hand. The bread that feels heavier is more nutritious. Whole wheat flour is naturally heavier, firmer, and more nutrient dense than airy white bread.

parent power-ade

We can give our kids what they need no matter where they eat outside our homes. When they're with us, we can replenish their reserves, balance out their nutrients, and give them the energy they need to go back out there another day. We already make so many choices in their best interest. We carefully choose many aspects of their lives until they go out on their own. We choose the neighborhood in which they live. We choose their friends when they're very young. We choose their clothes until they have an opinion. We monitor how much television they watch and what video games they play. We teach them how to cross streets safely, how to ride bicycles with helmets, how not to talk to strangers. We show them how to take care of their bodies by brushing their teeth, washing with soap, and what to do if they get hurt. We do all this and yet pay little attention to what they eat and how it affects them. We even wrestle over which school to send them to beginning in preschool. These choices will have little impact if our children aren't prepared to take advantage of them.

Our children are all born with learning styles, preferences, strengths, and weaknesses. Just as we are all born with certain propensities toward disease or addictions, we don't have to succumb to these natural tendencies without a fight. If we can change our habits and improve our quality of life, then we can increase our children's odds of success by feeding them right.

Chapter 2

THe roLe of parents

The apple does not fall far from the tree.
DUTCH Proverb

Jenny lovingly pieced together her dinner: 2 ounces of beef, a three-bean salad, and Italian bread. She was finally starting to get the hang of this high-protein, low-carb diet. She had more energy than she'd had in years, and the pounds were melting off like the snow after a spring storm. But her children stared at their plates like they were covered with a variety of creepy crawlies.

"I never thought I'd say this, Mom, but are we ever going to have vegetables again?" said Josh, 14 years old and the best on his swim team.

"Do we get dessert tonight, Mom?" asked 6-year-old Susan as she moved the beans around her plate without eating one.

"I wonder where your father is," Jenny said without answering either one of their questions. "He's been late every night for the past 2 weeks."

Just then the sound of the garage door opening made them all sit perfectly silent and still. Daddy was home.

"Hey, hon, sorry I'm late. The meeting ran long, so I picked up dinner for us all on the way home," Steven said as he began to unpack a variety of sizes of bags and cartons and pushed aside the plates already on the table.

"But I already made dinner," Jenny said. "This is the third time you've brought dinner home this week. I never asked you to do that."

"Chinese food! Thanks, Dad," Josh said and began to shovel his beef and beans back into their serving bowls and filled his plate with chicken chow mein instead.

"Ooh, can I open my fortune cookie now?" Susan asked, already ripping open the plastic pouch.

"Well, you all eat what you want. I'm happy with the dinner I prepared for us," Jenny said and tearfully began to spoon some three-bean salad into her mouth.

"Don't take it personally, Jen," Steven began. "It's just that your diet doesn't sit right in my body. The gas I get could shoot a rocket into space!"

Jenny smiled. She knew he was right. Maybe she could make some changes that would meet all of their needs and not just hers. But that just seems like so much work. She didn't even know what a 6-year-old, a 14-year-old, and a 40-year-old man needed in their diets.

I'm a Parent, not a nutritionist!

Mealtime mayhem begins within an hour of a child's birth. Whether you chose to breastfeed or bottle-feed your infant, the hospital nursing staff had something to say about how, when, and how much. Those of us who thought we were prepared for this scenario soon found ourselves doubting our authority as parents, even if we could only count our experience in hours, not years. Nurses and even pediatricians contradict our feeding philosophies, and unless we're quite strong-willed, we allow them to make the decision of how to feed our child instead. And we wonder if maybe they do know best.

But health care workers aren't the only ones. Before you know it, you bend to the wills of well-intentioned friends and family members all anxious to advise you on what and how your child should eat. Maybe they know more than we do. And then come the media. Food commercials bombard you with "what kids love" or "what choosy moms choose" or "fun food for finicky eaters." Maybe they have an inside track into what's good for kids. Then there's school. School breakfast and lunch programs proclaim "adequate nutrition" for all children. Maybe they should eat two of their three meals at school. Maybe "adequate" is good enough.

But you don't need a degree in nutrition to know what's good for your kids. You know them better than any doctor. You love them more than any family or friends (even grandparents). You have a higher stake in their future than any media conglomerate or school. You are more than capable to feed your kids right, and you can do a better job than "adequate." It's time to take back the controls. It's time to find out what your children need in order to perform at their best, now and in the future.

THE BROCCOLI STOPS HERE!

As much as we all believe that nutrition is important, acting responsibly according to that belief is a different story. Accepting responsibility for your family's nutrition can be intimidating. Your decisions will not always be popular. You'll have to take more time out of your already busy day to make nutrition a consideration. And sometimes you'll fail miserably and cave into the temptations of picking up fast food, skipping breakfast, or buying a lot of processed packaged foods at the grocery store. Yes, this is an awesome responsibility, but you're up to it. After all, you are the grown-up.

Kids will always push your limits and test your resolve. They know how much whining will get them what they want; they know how long to push those peas around their plates without eating them before you give up trying to get them to eat them; they know just what to say to make you feel like the world's worst parent who doesn't really love them because you won't buy them chocolate peanut butter cereal every week. Kids aren't stupid. But you're smarter! You know what's best. You know what foods make them hyper, what foods make their stomachs gurgle too much, and what foods seem to help them stay balanced or focused. You are more than capable to make nutrition decisions on behalf of your kids. Kids like structure and perform better within a defined set of boundaries. So it is with eating. You can create the structure and define the boundaries for them. Don't worry—there will still be plenty of room for creativity and choice.

Take a Whole Look at "Wheat"

Bread marketers know that consumers believe "wheat" to be healthier than white. So they use terms like *wheat bread* and *multigrain* to attract buyers to breads that are mostly made of refined flour. Choose breads, cereals, and other grains that say "whole wheat" or "whole grain."

From the very beginning, moms have been charged with safeguarding their families' nutritional health. Although more of us work outside the home than ever before, our traditional role has changed very little. We maintain such a hectic pace, with tighter and tighter schedules, that meeting the demands of our role as nutritional gatekeeper for our families seems overwhelming. After a long, exhausting day at work, many of us feel we simply don't have the time or energy to prepare delicious, nutritious meals or to supervise our kids' eating habits. But we have a unique opportunity—and a responsibility—to teach our children about the benefits of sound nutrition.

Before you can teach your kids about good nutrition, you need to first educate yourself. A recent U.S. Department of Agriculture study found that the more a mom knows about nutrition, the less likely her children are to be overweight. The good habits you put into your children now will follow them into their adulthoods and into the lives of your grandchildren. If you grew up in a nutritionally challenged home, you can break the cycle of poor eating habits with your own families. Knowledge is power, and now you have that power.

Which Comes First, the Chicken or the Egg?

The amount of DHA in a mother's breast milk depends on the amount of DHA in her diet. Infants nursing from mothers who had higher levels of DHA in their diets also had better mental development at 1 year of age.

SHOW anD TeLL

For better or for worse, we are the greatest influence in our children's lives. They learn more from what they see us do than what we tell them to do. Remember show and tell time in school? Kids came to school with treasures cupped in their hands to show their classmates. Everyone watched carefully. They couldn't wait to see what their friend brought to show. They could care less about what they had to say about it. The power is in the show. We are the show. We are their primary role models. By what you bought at the grocery store, what you served for meals, and what you yourself ate today, what did you *show* your children about nutrition? What a sobering thought!

As the most influential people in a child's life, parents set the stage for childhood eating habits. Whether you realize it or not, you are in the spotlight giving your kids a steady stream of information about when, what, and how much to eat. A parent's level of physical activity correlates to children's physical activity. Children of active parents are roughly six times more likely to be physically active than kids whose parents are card-carrying couch potatoes. Since nutrition and exercise go hand in hand, it's important to note the influence our own habits of both have on our kids.

DOES HEREDITY PLAY A ROLE?

Heredity plays a role in that kids of obese parents have a greater chance at becoming obese themselves, but for the more common situations of poor eating habits, heredity (or genetics) doesn't have an influence. Ironically, even those children whose parents are obese are only partly at risk because of their genes. Parental modeling of both eating and exercise has just as much influence. Kids with low energy may be born that way, but today's lifestyles only make the problems worse. The average American child spends several hours every day watching television or playing video games—time that in previous years might have been spent playing outside or doing something else more physical. It's not that they don't expend energy while viewing; it's that they eat high-calorie snacks *while* they're viewing. You may have the cards stacked against you because of heredity, but in the end your parent card trumps the rest.

Gut Feelings

Take your cues from your intestines. The intestinal lining and muscular walls are richly supplied with nerves, referred to as the "gut brains." They react to emotions as well as foods, which is why stress can give you indigestion or stomach pains.

FOOD POLICE: HOW TO MONITOR WHAT YOUR CHILD EATS, WHERE, AND WHEN

Now that you're convinced that you do indeed have the power to make a positive impact on your children's eating habits and nutrition, how vigilant do you need to be about it? Yes, you'll prepare the meals you eat together as well as their lunches to eat at school, but how tight of a rein do you need to have on your kids? After all, you can't be with them all the time. And unless you have spies, you just have to hope for the best when they eat away from home. Is it completely up to us to make sure our kids always eat right? At what point will they take responsibility for themselves?

There are ways to be involved without smothering your child. You can be involved directly by going over the school menus together and making wise choices at the beginning of the week. You can make sure that what you have in your refrigerator and pantry are the right foods, so that if your kids make food choices when you're not around, they at least have the right foods to choose from. You can ask them what they ate for dinner at a friend's house in case they tried something new that they liked. That way you can offer to make it at home sometime, and they won't think you are just checking up on them.

You can get more involved indirectly by joining a parent group at school that monitors what is served in the lunchroom. You can encourage your kids to invite their friends over, so that you are the one who provides the snacks for all of them. More than just your child benefits from this hospitality. You can volunteer to bring in food for a special occasion at school, whether it is a holiday party or something connected to what the kids are studying, like other cultures or languages.

You won't be able to control every aspect of your child's eating, and at some point kids will take on the responsibility themselves. They will rely on the habits we set now when they're ready. Vicki's teenage son, Charles, made her smile when at 14 he told her what day of the week he wanted to buy lunch at school (he was allowed to buy only once a week). "I'm going to buy on Wednesday. It looks like they make a great chicken Caesar salad," he said. "And it's huge! At least I know there'll be enough protein in it to get me through until dinner." This came after years of going over the weekly school lunch menus and critically looking at the nutritional values of the offerings. To Charles this is now a normal part of life, and at 14 he is finally beginning to put into practice himself what his parents taught him. The goal is to eventually hand the responsibility over to our kids when they're ready. But for now it's quite appropriate for you to hold onto as much of it as possible.

Why Not White?

Even though white is typically a symbol of purity, when it comes to the nutritional value of foods, white has been blackened. This is mostly true of those foods that are processed or manmade. White flour and white rice have been processed white. The most nutritious part of these foods, the bran content or brown color, has been bleached out for looks. Even a naturally white potato is less nutrient dense than its cousin the sweet potato, which is yellow or orange in color. To get your children to appreciate the nutrient value of foods, teach them that colorful foods are healthy foods.

DON'T GIVE UP—DON'T GIVE IN!

It is so tempting when you encounter resistance to back off or give up. Most of us will have to make some major changes in our buying, preparation, and eating habits if we're going to provide our families both nutritious and delicious foods. Those changes may not always go over smoothly with the very people we're trying to serve. But that's OK. They don't have to understand or even agree with what's for dinner. Don't let grumbling, whining, or refusal to eat get in your way. Kids will eat when they're hungry, and when they're hungry enough, they'll eat whatever is available. All you have to do is make sure the right things are available. In the case of nutrition, the path of least resistance is the path to obesity, a sedentary lifestyle, sugar-related syndromes, diseases and illnesses, poor growth, pediatric hypertension, tooth decay, and a host of learning problems.

Not from Concentrate

When this label appears on a fruit juice package, many consumers believe it means a nutritionally superior juice. Not necessarily so. "Concentrated" simply means that the water has been removed, and the consumer adds it back in before drinking. The juice you buy that is not from concentrate may contain more vitamin C than "made from concentrate" juice. Of course the juice you squeeze at home is always most nutritious, since it has not been processed in any way.

model moderation

Making all out changes to how your family eats may be cause for protest, but remember you can't change everything at the same time. Take small bites out of this challenge to change how your family eats and give them a chance to adjust. Accept that this is not a perfect process, nor should it be. Individual needs, tastes, and preferences should always be taken into account. Try not to get caught up in an all-or-nothing approach. Some days will be better than others. Some days your kids will eat what you prepare, and other days they just won't.

Every family and each child in every family has its own nutritional needs and challenges. Instead of looking at what your child ate at one meal, look at their overall eating for a week instead. *Everything in moderation*. Remove the words *never* and *always* from your vocabulary. Replace them with *sometimes* and *once in a while*. Sometimes you can go to a fast-food restaurant. Once in a while you can have cookies for a snack. Sometimes you can buy lunch at school. Once in a while you can have soda with dinner. Model moderation, and no one in your family will mistake you for a nutrition Nazi.

we're in this together

Families may consist of individuals, but in reality they are one unit. We need to act like a team by planning together, preparing together, and playing together. But every team has a captain, and you are the captain of your team. This way you model cooperation and leadership. Effective leaders are very in tune with the needs of those who follow them. See yourself as a servant leader—one who puts the needs of others above your own.

Take the lead by inviting everyone in the family to plan the menus for the coming week. A great way to keep track of a recipe that everyone loves is to tape a piece of paper inside an often-used cupboard and write down your favorite meals. If you find yourselves at a loss for what to have for dinner, someone can look down the list and make a suggestion everyone will love. Post the week's menu where everyone can see it. That way no one will be surprised that Thursday is meatloaf night. Have your kids go through the refrigerator and pantry and tell you what staples you need to buy that week. Are we out of milk? Do we need bread? Is there enough juice for the week? Not only will this approach help make list making more efficient, but it offers even a 4-year-old the chance to contribute. Include the whole family in meal planning, and you cut down on complaints later.

Good preparation equals success. You have to do your homework if you're going to pass the test. Kids of all ages can help in meal preparation. Vicki's husband, Chip, took their two boys to the grocery store with him every week from the day they were born. As teenagers they now know how to find what's on the list in the store, compare unit pricing, and put the food away when they return home.

In the kitchen, kids can help if you let them. Get them into the action. Let them help choose the food, but instead of asking "What vegetable do you want tonight?" ask, "Should we have green beans or corn?" This offers them a choice without giving them full reign. If you have older children who are competent in the kitchen, assign them one night of the week to prepare the family meal. A little responsibility can go a long way. They will have to plan the menu and put on the grocery list the ingredients they require. They will have to plan ahead to make sure dinner gets to the table on time.

How about an after-dinner walk or bike ride? Be the leader in this and suggest a way to get moving together. You're not training for a marathon, just looking for ways to stay active and model that value to your kids. You'll be surprised at the conversations that begin when you walk together. It's good for the body and the mind. Sometimes take the activity inside and have your own dinner and a movie night. There's nothing wrong with pulling the tray tables out and sitting them beside the couch in front of the television as long as you're doing it together. Plan a particularly special menu for movie night. This is a great opportunity to let your kids call the shots on this one. If you make it a regular part of your routine, this night may become your family's favorite.

Sweet Breads

Even the best breads contain a bit of sweetener, such as sugar, honey, molasses, or fructose. Sugar makes the bread tender and helps the crust to brown. Don't be a sweetener purist when it comes to bread; you'll end up with a mouthful of dry, tasteless grain. The same is true for salt. Salt adds flavor and helps the bread to rise. A pinch of salt and a bit of sweetener are necessary to get the bread just right.

Most of us are completely capable of feeding our own children right, but we've been brainwashed to believe that only the experts know. Obstacles threaten to distract us from our desire to make nutrition a priority. Convenience screams for our attention, and we find ourselves more dependent on the schools to feed our kids than we should. But you have more power than you think. Each day you have choices: to plan or not to plan; to pack a lunch or let them buy; to monitor what they eat or ignore; to ask questions or remain ignorant. Parents make all the difference when it comes to what kids eat, whether your own hands prepared it or someone else's did. Control what you can control, and instill the good nutritional habits. Model the right choices. After that, you can relax in the fact that you're setting your child up for success.

PART II

GROWING BODIES/ GROWING MINDS

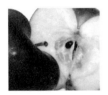 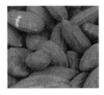 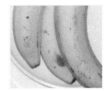

Chapter 3

1- TO 3-year-OLDS

*It's bizarre that the produce manager is more important
to my children's health than the pediatrician.*

meryl streep

"What is it now?" Brenda asked her already-overstimulated and over-tired 2½-year-old. Scott just couldn't seem to play nicely today.

"Mom, Scott hit Brianna again," her 5-year-old tattled.

Brianna, almost 3, sat on the leaf-littered grass crying. Her mother, Brenda's best friend, Sandy, ran over to soothe her daughter once again.

"I'm sorry," Brenda said to Sandy. "I just don't know what's gotten into him today."

"It's OK," Sandy said. "Hey, we're heading out to Burger World for lunch. Do you want to come?"

Lunch. Brenda hadn't even realized it was that time. She'd fed the kids breakfast 6 hours ago! It was at that moment that Brenda understood why Scott was so out of sorts. The only thing he'd eaten that day was a blueberry Pop Tart, juice, and a handful of oat cereal mid-morning. As appealing as eating out sounded, Brenda knew better. A much bigger eruption brewed beneath the surface of her son's demeanor. They had to go home—and now!

"Thanks, Sandy," Brenda said. "But we'll have to take a rain check."

Brenda plucked Scott off the ground and onto her hip then hurried her harried children into their van. She slammed the door, shutting out the tantrums that resulted from their quick retreat. At least if they were going to fall apart, they might as well all do it at home.

Who knew we'd long for the days when our babies sat safely in our laps? Now all they do is move—under us, over us, around us, and away from us! Vicki's firstborn was 18 months old when he walked away from her in a department store and hid among the ladies' lingerie. As exciting as it is to witness the physical, mental, and social milestones our little ones are reaching, it's a bittersweet stage. When they were babies, we fed them by either bottle or breast and spooned them puree from baby food jars. It was prepackaged, easy to buy, easy to use, and easy to remember.

Now they want to eat standing up. They want to use their hands and do it themselves. They have more food preferences than just not wanting to eat mashed squash. They choose food by what they can pick up between their cute little fingers, what it feels like in their mouth, and basically just by the way it looks. The challenges don't end there. Scheduled eating is just as important now as it was when they were infants. If you didn't schedule your baby, you may find that finding ways to feed your toddler is a hair-pulling challenge.

One for the Money

It's time to transition from baby food to regular table food. Believe it or not, your food bill will drop dramatically. Jar food and formula is expensive, so rejoice in the fact that your child can now eat what you cook for dinner—with some modifications. There are a couple of obstacles to pleasurable mealtimes at this stage. Teething is still a major factor and can hinder your progress at introducing new and exciting foods. Be sensitive to the fact that sometimes chewing hurts even if it's just applesauce. Right now your precious one is fast becoming a social butterfly. As enjoyable as that is, they can then become easily distracted. If Grandma is visiting, your child may spend most of dinner time making eyes at her instead of eating. And even though you're elated about feeding table food, it's important to prepare meals with no added sugar or salt. In the long run what's good for your 1-year-old is good for the whole family. You may start saving on grocery money, but costs increase with loss of time and convenience.

Two for the Show

Two-year-olds are like adults who've recently gone through assertiveness training—they know what they want, and they don't hesitate to ask for it. Personality and temperament may dictate *how* they let you know, but the word *no* is now the most commonly used word in their growing vocabulary.

The "terrible twos" is a misnomer. The strong-willed child may challenge you anywhere between 18 months and 3 years, and eating becomes a battleground. Suddenly she notices what's on the shelves in the grocery store. Little hands reach for brightly wrapped goodies while you're in the check-out line. They see—they want.

Take advantage of this attraction by having some fun with food preparation. Use cookie cutters to create shapes out of their sandwiches. Offer variety in color and texture. Experiment with different breads and condiments. At this stage Vicki's boys loved "dip." Ketchup, mustard, ranch dressing, and even hot sauce were squeezed onto their plates for tasting. Have different fruits and veggies cut up on a plate where they can reach it or at least see it. Just as a painter works from a color-filled palette, our kids can develop their palette from the foods we offer. New experiences create new connections in the brain. The idea is to create as many connections as possible, so get creative with your food offerings.

Three to Get Ready

Meltdowns—they happen at home, at play group, in the store, on the playground, and most often right before dinner. Our mom called the time between 4:00 and 5:00 P.M. the "insanity hour." Toss into the mix a 3-year-old who's just beginning to get a handle on the English language (if it is your first language), knows how to ask for what he wants, but still can't temper the emotions that rule him. When they're hungry, they're hungry, and they want to eat right *now*. Even with an ever-increasing vocabulary, he still resorts to whining. Tolerance and patience are lost on a little one whose blood sugar is too low and can't explain to you that his tummy or head hurts just because he's hungry. You can encourage him to "use his words," but a better approach is to try to prevent the outbursts by feeding him nutrient-rich foods often. Their tummies are only about the size of their little fists, so give them a fistful of something that will stick with them every few hours. Avoid handfuls of sugar cereal or candy. Offer your little tot raisins or cheese or peanut butter crackers instead. It doesn't have to be the "best" food choice, but it shouldn't be the worst, either.

Why Won't They Sleep?

If you give your child something to eat right before bed or during the night, then her body is geared up for digestion and not geared down for sleep. Toddlers' tummies are no longer linked to sleep. We're past the point of falling asleep while nursing or waking to a wail of hunger. Even if *you* find yourself wanting a midnight snack, avoid modeling that behavior for your little one. If you've already created a monster with this habit, slowly but surely wean her off of the promise of food before sleep or in the middle of the night. The bottom line is that food is a stimulant, and a body in motion is definitely not a body at rest. Replace eating with bedtime rituals that soothe the soul and tell the body and mind to slow down and not restart. Create a peaceful environment the hour before bedtime with a warm bath, a story, a lullaby, or prayers. The habits you create now follow them right into adulthood, so choose wisely. Set them up for a good night's sleep, and you'll all be ready for a good morning.

The Potty

Kids ultimately potty-train themselves. They're ready when they're ready, but we're usually ready long before they are. What and when we feed them can help or hinder their progress to wearing big boy or big girl underwear and staying dry and accident-free. We can set them up for success by giving them plenty of water to drink (preferable over juice or soda), making sure they eat enough fiber (peas, whole grain breads, blueberries, strawberries, baked beans, dried fruits, sweet white corn, peanuts, sunflower seeds, natural fruit juices/nectar mixed into shakes or smoothies), and eating at regular intervals so that their insides move more regularly. Avoid those foods and drinks that either make kids "go" too often or not often enough. Toddlers don't understand how or why their bodies work the way they do, but we can still talk to them about it. Help build their understanding by telling them that water makes the food move better inside their tummies and then out into the potty. Explain to them which foods are helper foods and which are not. They will grow in understanding as their digestive system grows. If your child still struggles with anything associated with potty training, consult your pediatrician.

Tough Teeth

Tooth decay can start as early as age 1. Have you ever seen an almost 3-year-old walking around with a baby bottle of milk or juice hanging from her mouth as a necessary accessory? Have you ever or been tempted to put your child to bed with a bottle? Baby bottle tooth decay or bottle rot can be very destructive to your child's baby teeth and eating habits. Acid found in the sugars in milk, fruit juice, vitamins, and formula dissolve the tooth and cause decay. Kids' teeth can appear normal and then change their appearance within weeks. Kids who develop this infection have a greater chance of continuing to get decay with every emerging baby tooth and an increased chance of tooth decay in their adult teeth. Painful abscesses, cavities, missing teeth, and pediatric dental work (usually gum surgery or tooth pulling) can easily compromise eating.

Good dental hygiene begins with the first tooth. You'll need to change your toddler's eating and drinking habits if you want to prevent this uncomfortable and unpleasant problem. Avoid giving a bottle in the crib to get your child to sleep. And remember to clean her mouth after feedings. Make sure juices in bottles are diluted, and make the switch to only water as soon as you comfortably can. If your child's already in pain, offer finger foods at mealtime. If she uses a spoon, make sure it is rubber coated so contact with swollen gums or sensitive teeth isn't as painful. Yes, the baby teeth will fall out, but if they fall out too soon it affects how well the adult teeth come in. Take care of it now, or you'll be paying an orthodontist by age 9.

Eating in Bits and Bites

Abraham Lincoln said, "Little by little does the trick." That's how a toddler eats—little by little. He may turn his nose up to your sensibly prepared, nutritious meal in favor of eating cheese and peanut butter on bread four times a day. Kids at this age are picky at best and distressing at worst. Try not to take the rejection of your cuisine personally. Their development is to blame, not your cooking. As important as it is to help them eat with and like the rest of the family, you just shouldn't count on it right now. There's nothing wrong with grazing as long as you make every bite count. Make nutrient-rich foods like avocados, pasta, broccoli, peanut butter, brown rice and other grains, potatoes, cheese, poultry, eggs, squash, fish, sweet potatoes, kidney beans, tofu, and yogurt available and within reach. Getting them to try new foods is a good place to start, but don't be surprised if they eat a plateful of broccoli one day and completely reject it on another.

A great way to negotiate trying of new foods is to tell them they need to eat as many bites as they are old. A 3-year-old needs to try and eat *three* bites (no matter how small). The key to getting through this phase is to offer variety in small portions. Relax and remember—little by little, this too shall pass.

Fish and Flax

Your skin may reflect a fatty acid deficiency if it is dry, flakey, and has an unhealthy look. Try adding flax oil, tuna, and salmon to your diet a few times a week. After a few months of eating these foods high in essential fatty acids, your skin will look healthier and feel smoother.

Baby on the Run!

On your mark, get set, go! Toddlers don't really "toddle." They run, jump, and climb on, around, and over anything in their path. They are in constant motion. And even though the average 1-year-old has tripled the birthweight, toddlers gain weight more slowly. They burn more calories than they consume. They don't seem to sit still for anything, even food. They are explorers who won't be bothered with a sit-down feast. The good news is that they are doing a great job building muscle strength and flexibility. The bad news is that we must be more diligent in our efforts to pack nutrition into every little bite they take. Toddlers need enough protein to ensure both physical growth and brain function. They need fat for energy and normal brain growth. Try to combine both in every meal when possible. Your toddler's energy level will keep you hopping. Just make sure he's never running on empty.

Juice Abuse

"I want juice!"

"Try some water, honey."

"No. Juice!"

Sound familiar? Toddlers don't really *need* juice. Limit juice so your child will have an appetite for more nutritious foods throughout the day. Too much juice can also cause "failure to thrive" in little ones. It can also cause diarrhea because some of the sugars in fruit juice aren't completely absorbed from the gastrointestinal tract into the bloodstream.

How do you combat juice abuse? Give them water instead. The idea is to hydrate children. In hot weather, don't reach for the juice; give them a water bottle. Young children get easily overheated and dehydrated if you're not on guard, so carry pint-sized bottles of water for your pint-sized cutie. Even if you live in a cold climate, your child's at risk for dehydration. When we heat our homes, we lose much-needed moisture. Just make sure everyone reaches for water first when they're thirsty. Water helps everything run smoother—it's like greasing the wheels of our brain.

Got Milk?

Do you wonder about giving your kids soda, coffee, tea, or energy drinks? They have no place in a tot's diet. When in doubt, choose milk instead. If your child won't drink milk by itself, add some chocolate or vanilla syrup to make a tasty treat. Add milk with other ingredients in a blender to make a shake or smoothie. Milk is still milk, even if it's all mixed up with ice cream and fruit! The benefits of milk outweigh the small amount of sweeteners added to make it more appealing. Children need milk in order to get enough calcium and vitamin D. Form good milk-drinking habits early on, so your child will form dense bones later.

Do I Need to Give My Child a Vitamin?

It depends. As a general rule, toddlers who eat reasonably healthy diets do not need added vitamins. If they eat whole foods (fresh vegetables, fresh fruit, whole grains, etc.), then they will get the necessary vitamins in the healthiest way. Even though there are times when they are picky eaters, they'll get their vitamin requirements from the foods consumed.

Unfortunately, since more and more of our foods are highly processed in a way that minimizes their vitamin and mineral contents, it wouldn't hurt to give kids a multivitamin as a supplement. At some point they will eat a more balanced diet, so it's really a matter of providing a vitamin "safety net" if you're struggling to get your child to eat right. Keep in mind that vitamins should also be taken in moderation—more is not better!

Picky Eaters Are Made, Not Born

What you like to eat affects what your kids eat. Just because you don't like apples doesn't mean you can't offer them to your kids. Kelly stopped buying tomatoes because her husband didn't like them. Without realizing it, she taught her kids not to "like" them or even taste them, for that matter. Picky eaters aren't born; they're taught. Offer a variety of foods, even if they're not *your* favorites. Kids eat what's around them, so if you fill the cupboards with cookies and high-sugar cereal, that's what they'll eat. Try to load your fridge with fresh, cut-up veggies and dips; top the counter with colorful fruits and mixed nuts; give kids the opportunity to grab a handful of grapes instead of a bag of chips.

Part of being picky lies in the fact that toddlers want to exercise their independence. They may say no to something just because they can. Just make sure that their choices are nutritious, and it won't matter if they say yes or no.

Sweet Treats

It's not necessary to cut out sugar all together from a toddler's diet. Naturally sweet foods such as fruit and some vegetables pose no harm to a young child's diet. On the other hand, cookies, candies, and cakes that are high in sugars should not make up a major part of a child's diet. These "treat" foods not only contain sugar but are low in other nutrients. When kids eat a lot of high-sugar foods, they crave more of the same. This sugar cycle cuts down drastically on their nutrient intake. Filling themselves up with "goodies" leaves their tiny bellies too full and their appetite too low to then try to eat other, more nutritious foods. These "treats" are made up of simple sugars that enter the bloodstream quickly. A "sugar high" rises and then drops quickly, causing difficult to manage mood swings. Children are more sensitive to the effects of simple sugars because of their small size and immature body systems.

Annoying Allergies

Even though kids are exposed to cold germs every day, their chronic stuffy nose or ear infections might be a sign of allergies. Allergies affect the lives of millions of people around the world. Fresh spring flowers, a friend's cat or dog, even dust can make people itch, sneeze, and scratch. But what about that seemingly innocent peanut butter sandwich, glass of milk, or fish fillet?

A food allergy is a reaction of the body's immune system to something in a food, most often a protein. Food allergy symptoms generally occur within minutes to hours of eating the offending food and include swelling and itching of the throat, nausea, and skin rashes. Some or all of these symptoms may be present and at varying degrees of severity. The eight most common food allergens are milk, eggs, peanuts, tree nuts, soy, wheat, fish, and shellfish. Many other foods have also been identified as allergens for some people. Most people don't have a food allergy when they have a reaction; they're experiencing a food sensitivity or intolerance to a certain food instead.

The first step in treatment is to avoid the offending food or ingredient. Substitute the allergen food with other nonoffending proteins whenever possible to maintain a balanced diet. In some cases, medication will still be needed to regulate severe reactions. If you suspect your child has a true food allergy, you should see an allergist and dietitian for diagnosis and treatment options.

Fats and Fiber

Because fiber gives you a sense of fullness sooner, eating a fiber-filled meal is likely to prompt you to eat less fat. Hence, too little fiber may make you eat more fat for fullness.

Are Organics Worth It?

Supposedly government standards keep all foods and drinks safe, but many doctors and researchers recommend organics because they're produced without harsh pesticides, artificial hormones, or antibiotics. Since a toddler's system can't tolerate the use of these things, a good rule of thumb is to choose organic versions of things your kids eat all the time.

Yes, organic foods can be more expensive, so which are worth buying? Fruits and veggies (especially apples, bell peppers, celery, cherries, imported grapes, nectarines, peaches, pears, potatoes, red raspberries, spinach, and strawberries) are definitely worth buying organic. If your child is a heavy drinker of 100 percent fruit juice, adores applesauce, and munches regularly on dried fruits, consider buying organic. Even though the amount of pesticides is lower, kids who consume large quantities of any of these are at risk. Meat, dairy, and eggs are worth buying organic if your child eats a lot of nitrate-heavy meats like hot dogs and deli meats. Breads, cereals, and pasta have much lower pesticide residue and are not necessarily worth buying organic.

If you choose not to buy organic, you can help lighten the risks associated with pesticides by washing produce thoroughly and by choosing skim or low-fat milk and lean meats.

Edible Energy

The food guide pyramid suggests a low-fat, high-fiber diet. You can offer a less restrictive diet for your children without making an entirely separate meal for them. Controlling their portions, increasing their milk, and adding good fats at mealtimes are the most effective ways to adjust the pyramid to fit the needs of your toddler. The following portion sizes are appropriate:

Calcium—for growing bones and brains: 500 milligrams (equal to 16 ounces milk daily or 1 cup milk and ½ cup yogurt with ½ cup broccoli)

Fruit juice—for a sweet treat: 10 ounces (equal to 1½ cups pure fruit juice or 1 cup juice and 1 Popsicle)

Iron—for steady energy: 10 milligrams (¼ cup raisins or whole grain cereal, 3 ounces fish, or ½ cup green leafy vegetables)

Zinc—for a strong immune system: 10 milligrams (3 ounces of red meat or poultry or ½ cup beans/nuts or fortified cereals)

Fat-soluble vitamins—for growth and overall health:

Vitamin D (found in 1 cup of dairy products; milk, yogurt, cheese)

Vitamin A (found in yellow/orange vegetables; carrots, squash)

Vitamin C (found in many citrus fruits such as oranges; asparagus; peas; strawberries)

THE TODDLER BRAIN

A brain-healthy diet consists of nutrition *and* exercise. Our brains need a workout as much as our bodies do. Even though our toddlers are in constant motion, their brains may be couch potatoes. Over the course of a week, try to incorporate the following exercises that promote connection between mind and body. Aligned to an effective workout routine, these mental calisthenics can go a long way to improve brain function by preparing it to accept learning opportunities more easily.

Heads, Shoulders, Knees, and Toes

This is a great way to warm up both your toddler's mind and body. This classic game works on both gross motor skills and cognitive skills. Do it with your child as part of a daily warm-up. Add other body parts to stretch your child more as time goes on.

Head and shoulders, knees and toes, knees and toes,
(touch each corresponding body part)
Head and shoulders, knees and toes, knees and toes,
(touch each corresponding body part)
Eyes and ears and mouth and nose,
(touch each corresponding body part)
Head and shoulders, knees and toes, knees and toes!
(touch each corresponding body part)

The Cow Goes . . .

Help your child identify what she hears and its name, and you go a long way to making those all important brain connections. Start with what children already know: animal sounds that they hear often; vehicles like trucks, ambulances, fire trucks, airplanes, and so forth; home sounds like the doorbell, a door opening or closing, the telephone, and more. Then, to create new connections, introduce new sounds by either creating them yourself or taking them somewhere where they will hear them.

Who Is It?

Kids at this age still love faces. Spend some time helping them learn the names of people they know and those people they don't see regularly. Go through your photo albums or photos you might have on your refrigerator with them and see how many people they can name. They may need some prompting like "Where's Uncle Chad?" or "I see Daddy. Do you see Daddy?"

Over time they will be able to quickly identify even those relatives they only see once a year. This also helps develop their speaking skills. Have them repeat the names to you. Eventually they will be able to say them without prompting and say them correctly.

Do It with Dough

Homemade play dough is easy and inexpensive to make and store. As a toddler's fine motor skills develop, so too does his desire to create.

You can add food coloring to different dough batches to give your child a rainbow of choices to work with. Just make sure his fingers stay in the dough and not in his mouth!

Materials
4 cups flour
1 cup salt
1¾ cups water
Mixing bowl
Red, blue, yellow, and green food coloring
Fun tools like plastic silverware, rolling pin, and cookie cutters

Directions
1. Mix flour, salt, and water in a bowl to make dough; knead with your hands until the dough is well blended.
2. Divide dough into four parts and add desired food coloring to each. Knead until color is well blended.
3. Store in an airtight container.
4. Encourage kids to explore the dough with the tools provided. If they want to use something else, let them.

To Touch You Is to Know You

Toddlers still want to touch everything in order to understand it. Unfortunately, as parents we spend a lot of time telling them what *not* to touch. Let's give them some much-needed opportunities to explore their sense of touch safely. Fill each of four to six paper bags with an item that has an interesting texture. Something smooth could be a rubber ball. Something rough could be sandpaper. Something soft could be a favorite stuffed toy. Something hard could be a block. Be sure the items in the bags are safe to touch with no sharp points.

Have your child stick her hand into the bag without looking inside. Ask her what it feels like. If she has trouble verbalizing, suggest, "Is it soft?" Once your child identifies the texture, have her guess what the item is.

Sit Time

Our kids rarely find time to sit still unless we find the time for them. Being able to sit still and listen will make the transition to a preschool and later a traditional school setting more pleasurable for both your child and the teacher. Sitting in front of the television is not "sit time." Up until this point you are probably reading with your child on a regular basis. Your child is sitting and listening, but it's time to take it a step further.

Choose a time of day when your child is well rested and fed. Tell him it is "sit time," place him on the couch or a comfy bean bag chair, and have him listen to either music or a book on tape with headphones on. Begin with 10 minutes. Over time work up to having your child sit and listen for 30–45 minutes at a time. There are plenty of listening choices from nursery rhyme tapes to their favorite story books on tape. You can rent these from your local library or buy them at a bookstore.

Some children may not like the feeling of the headphones on their ears and heads. Make sure that they are softly cushioned and fit well. They will get used to them and begin to look forward to their sit time. This activity transitions into silent reading time later on.

Chapter 4

4- TO 6-year-OLDS

*A food is not necessarily essential just
because your child hates it.*
katherine whitehorn

Anne sat in the school auditorium amazed at how quickly the year had passed. "Kindergarten is over!" she thought while watching Nate walk across the stage wearing a construction paper mortar board with a rainbow-colored yarn tassel. But that wasn't the only thing he wore. A scowl covered his face just as frequently as his beautiful smile used to. What's wrong now? He was fine this morning.

Nate left the procession to sit next to his mom and little sister. "I don't want to go to the park," he declared.

"But your whole class is going to the park for lunch," Anne reminded.

"I don't care. I want to eat lunch at home instead," he said.

Anne shook her head and led her children out to the parking lot and into their car. "I give up," she thought. "I never know what to expect with this kid anymore."

Halfway home Nate started to cry. You've got to be kidding! Now what?

"I want to go to the park!" he said through his sniffling and sobbing.

Anne made a U-turn and headed back toward the park. This was no surprise. The only thing she could count on was that Nate would change his mind.

The teacher had ordered lunch for everyone. Anne remembered filling out the form indicating which sandwich Nate wanted—turkey or tuna. He chose tuna. Anne looked at her son now, sitting on a picnic blanket on the soft grass, and her heart fell. There's that scowl again.

"I don't want tuna," Nate said. "I want turkey."

"You ordered tuna, Nate. You have tuna. Just eat it," Anne said in her most parental voice.

"But I don't want tuna!" Nate burst into tears once again, and once again Anne led him to the car.

"We'll eat at home. And I won't change my mind!" she said strapping him into his car seat. "If you can't make a decision, I'll make it for you."

Anne hated being a dictator. Shouldn't she give Nate choices? "If he could make up his mind, I guess it would work," she thought.

WHAT TO EXPECT NOW

Look out, here we come—no longer a babe in any way, shape, or form. Four- to 6-year-olds are definitely kids now. When they sleep, you see how long and stretched out their bodies are on the bed. The chubby cheeks of baby fat have disappeared, leaving a more defined look. Their personalities are more established now. During the preschool and early school years, we see great increases in emotional, cognitive, and muscular development.

By age 4 or 5, most kids believe they are the center of their universe. They like to be in control, and even when they play with others they barter for that control. "I'll let you play with my train, if you let me play with your car." They can follow simple game rules, but they still get upset if they don't win. Five-year-olds like to pretend and imitate adult behavior. Take advantage of this tendency and show them how you choose and prepare foods. Curiosity is their strong trait, and now is a great time to explain the how's and why's behind why we eat what we eat. Kids at this age also choose their own friends now (usually same sex) and by 6 pair up with a "best" friend.

Sixes have a hard time making up their minds. They are a bundle of contradictions. One moment they want chocolate ice cream only to change their mind a moment later to cookie dough. Stubbornness invades their personality, and the desire to do things their own way overshadows their desire to please Mom or Dad. Patience and a smile go a long way to quelling the frustrations that come with a 6.

By the end of this stage, kids explore many basic concepts like count-ing, the alphabet, sizes, shapes, and colors. Special interests and talents may begin to emerge like art or music or athletics that you can nurture by taking them to museums, libraries, concerts, or athletic events. Books are especially important now whether your child is reading or not. Expo-sure to and exploration of the world of books builds a lifetime love of reading. Children's understanding about things used every day like money, food, or gadgets around the house will help you explain the rea-son behind why we do what we do. Conversations about what they eat and why it's good or bad for them are better received at this age.

Persuading the Picky Eater

Are you worried your child isn't eating as much as he should? Keep in mind that kids can grow at normal rates even when they eat very little. He may have a smaller appetite or he may be a finicky eater and just not willing to even taste certain foods. Although frustrating, this behavior doesn't have to impair growth. Appetites and food preferences change as a child grows. One way to persuade him to try new foods or eat vegetables is to include new foods with foods he already likes. Try mixing peas with macaroni and cheese. Add bananas to oatmeal if he doesn't like hot cereal. Casseroles are a great way to introduce new tastes and textures. Vegetables can be hidden among noodles and cheese or sauce. Stews and soups are other ways to introduce new foods into his diet. Try to offer small servings of different foods each meal. Offer him foods from all the necessary food groups every day. He may not eat from each group every day, but he has the opportunity to try if it is available to him. Kids eat with their eyes, so make food look more inviting by using cookie cut-ters to turn a sandwich or pancake into fun shapes. Just remember to consider how he eats over the course of a week, not the course of a day. If you're ever in doubt about his growth, consult his pediatrician.

Mealtime Tug-of-War

"Mom, I don't like meatloaf!" Kathy said.

"Just try one bite. Use your ketchup dip; you like that," said Mom.

Upset and hungry, Kathy cried, "No. I want hot dogs!"

Frustrated and on the edge of yelling, Mom replied, "You will eat what is at the table! I will not make another meal just for you!"

It is important to give calm and consistent answers to tantrums about food preferences. Do not give in to whining about ice cream for breakfast or cookies with dinner. If you decide to offer alternatives, try healthy ones with a little creativity such as yogurt in an ice cream cone at breakfast or a slice of chocolate chip banana with dinner. Meals and snacks given in a relaxed manner and on a regular basis make for pleasant eating times. After some time, your consistency will pay off, your child will adapt, and fussing over foods will decrease.

"Eggs"-actly How Many?

Most moms complain they can't get their kids to eat breakfast. But in some households (like Kelly's), kids love breakfast-type foods, especially eggs. Cook 'em any way—scrambled, hard boiled, soft boiled, over easy, you name it; Kelly's children eat eggs. They'd eat them every morning if they could. But they can't. Kelly reminds them, "Too much of anything is just not good."

Eat Your Eggs

Because eggs are high in cholesterol, they are thought of as no-no's. Wrong! For most people who do not have high cholesterol or who are not sensitive to dietary cholesterol, consuming an egg a day won't significantly raise serum cholesterol levels. One egg three times a week can be part of a healthful diet.

How many eggs should a child eat each week? The American Heart Association recommends adults eat no more than three to four eggs each week, but it has no formal recommendations for children. Since an egg contains 213 milligrams of cholesterol, eating eggs too often can cause a diet high in cholesterol. However, eggs can be a healthy part of your child's diet in moderation. Eggs are high in protein, which kids need for muscular development, and they're high in iron, B vitamins, and minerals, which they need for steady energy levels.

Look at your child's overall eating plan. Try to balance her diet throughout the day and week. Since eggs are in the meat group, younger children should have two to six servings a day. Keep in mind eggs are found in many of the baked goods we eat and should be accounted for in the daily diet recommendations. The relationship between dietary cholesterol and blood cholesterol is controversial. Many dietitians believe it is more important to limit the amount of saturated fats in a person's diet than cholesterol.

LDL versus HDL

To remember the bad versus the good, think of LDL as "lousy" cholesterol, and HDL as "healthy" cholesterol.

Prepare to Test

Several things affect the accuracy of cholesterol blood tests. Fluctuations in weight, changes in diet, pregnancy, and excessive alcohol intake all wreak havoc on results. The most accurate results are obtained when your weight is stable for at least 2 weeks and you are eating your usual diet. While total cholesterol and HDL are fairly accurate without fasting, LDL is more accurate if obtained first thing in the morning after a 12-hour fast.

Lunch Duty

Once children reach kindergarten, they begin to take a bag lunch to school, sometimes prepared at the last minute or without much thought. Often they complain that they don't like "what Mom sends for lunch" or that they're "tired of peanut butter sandwiches." Since kids at this age begin to have their own preferences, it's a good time to involve them in selecting and preparing their lunch. Take time after dinner to make lunch together for the next day. Make sure there are plenty of good things to choose from, and then let your child put it together.

Lunch is important for replenishing nutrients already depleted from the morning's activities. Lunch is also a bridge to dinnertime. A lunch that isn't complete or eaten at all doesn't supply the adequate nutrients for brain and physical function required to sustain a child until dinner.

Try to mix proteins and carbohydrates (preferably not simple carbohydrates, like sugar) and make it kid-friendly. Cheese slices on whole wheat crackers with berries and yogurt is a well-balanced, simple-to-prepare, and easy-to-eat lunch for a young child. A bag lunch shouldn't be too big for your child's appetite or the time allowed for lunch. (In chapter 10 we give many meal suggestions for lunch at home or at school. Please refer to these meal plans and accompanying recipes for variety.)

The Meal Deal

Food preferences and peer pressure begin around age 4 or 5. As children begin eating away from home, they begin to see differences in how, when, and why to eat from their friends and other adults. As parents we need to continually offer healthy food choices whenever possible. Continue to talk openly with your child about foods and nutrients. By age 4, a child begins to understand consequences. You can explain "good" versus "bad" foods and why. She can now understand why sugar may cause her behavior to change in ways that may get her in trouble at school. Kids want to do the best they can, so it's up to us to provide them the tools they need to succeed.

The Cycle Starts Here

All children reap the benefit from the reduction of sugar in their diet as well as the increase of calcium found in milk at mealtimes, especially breakfast. Typically the most important meal of the day, breakfast is commonly overlooked because of busy morning schedules or tiredness. Getting yourself and your kids fed and ready and out the door (sometimes even before the sun rises) seems to be a miracle some days. It is tempting to hand your child a fruit-filled pastry or a sugar-filled breakfast bar to eat on the way to school, thinking "something is better than nothing." Unfortunately, not starting the day out right can lead to a domino effect throughout the day. Starting the day with a high amount of sugar most commonly found in our kids' favorite cereals and individually wrapped cereal bars adds to the difficulty parents and teachers have to keep kids on task or focused.

No Sweet Rewards

How many parents desperate to get broccoli into their preschooler promise candy for dessert if the veggies get eaten? This is an unwise nutritional bargain. It teaches children to dislike their veggies and value their sweets. Besides, when your child is older and on his own, who will stand beside him and encourage him to eat the good food first?

Stop the vicious cycle of sugar highs and lows, which exacerbates stress feelings and poor eating habits, which lead to impulsive behaviors and unwanted outbursts from our kids. Do yourselves and your kids a favor: start the day the right way. Try waking up 15 minutes earlier to allow time for a breakfast beyond that cereal bar. Actually, the time to mix up fruit, milk, and yogurt in a blender for a delicious smoothie takes far less than 15 minutes! Or prepare the night before some yogurt parfaits (see chapter 9). If your child loves breakfast meats such as sausage links or bacon, make them ahead of time and store in the fridge. A quick reheat is all you'll need in the morning for a protein-powered breakfast. Also try making whole wheat grain pancakes in advance and freezing them in storage bags; take out in the morning the amount needed, heat them up, and add a glass of milk. A little planning goes a long way.

Fiber for Kids

The skin on fruits provide a rich source of fiber. So, don't peel it away; instead, cut fruit into small easier-to-eat cubes or wedges. Serve fiber-rich juices with the true nectar rather than "pulp-free" versions.

Attention, Please

It's just before lunch at preschool.

"Michael, please come and sit in circle with the class," said Ms. Kelly. Michael came and sat down, all the while fidgeting on his carpet square, then calling out of turn, and finally backing up again at the block table.

"Michael, I said to join the group and sit still this time." Michael tried again. This time Ms. Kelly read a story. Although it only took 5 minutes to read, Michael left the circle before she finished. Frustrated, Ms. Kelly called to him once more.

"We are not finished yet, Michael. Please sit back down!"

Does Michael have ADHD, or is he undisciplined? It's hard to tell in this situation, but it's a common question from teachers to parents at this age. Constant fidgeting and an inability to concentrate don't necessarily mean a child needs medication. These can also be signs of immaturity or erratic blood sugar levels. The behavior still needs attention regardless of its root cause. Try to rule out behavior, maturity, and dietary causes first before reaching for the ADHD card. Your last stop should be your pediatrician, not the first.

We have unrealistic expectations of kids. We expect 4- and 5-year-olds who naturally have short attention spans, are hyperactive, and like to play to sit still for 3 hours or more at school without physical play time or a nutrient-rich snack when they need it. Experienced teachers with a background in early childhood development have great insight into what is appropriate at this age. If a teacher is struggling with your child, take the time now to investigate its cause so that the behavior doesn't follow your child into first, second, or third grade. Right now you have control over how your child's behavior is handled. Later on your choices will be few as the schools take more control. So check your parenting, check his health, and check your fridge. If you can't find the answer there, check with your pediatrician.

Presentation, Presentation!

It is all in the presentation when getting your picky eater to try something on the plate. Cutting sandwiches with cookie cutter shapes, making small pieces to eat with a toothpick, or arranging food on the plate to make a face are sure-fire ways to entice your youngster.

The Whole Fruit and Nothing but the Fruit

What happens when kids won't eat whole fruits but drink fruit juice instead? It was so much easier when all we had to do was open a baby food jar of peaches or pears or plums. Whether it's because whole fruits are more difficult to eat or their texture turns them away, some kids won't eat them. Parents think that if they just give their kids 100 percent real fruit juice, it replaces the need for whole fruits. Not so. Sugar found in fruit juice is still its primary ingredient, so there is little nutritional value to be found. Whole fruits *with* their skins (grapes, strawberries, apples, pears, etc.) provide us with vitamins and fiber, not just sugar. The American Association of Pediatrics recommends a limit of 4–6 ounces of 100 percent fruit juice. This is a *limit*, not a requirement. Your child does not *need* juice in her diet at all as long as she receives the nutrients from whole fruits and vegetables. Drinking too much juice can lead to poor eating habits, cavities, and overweight children.

There are some situations when 100 percent fruit juice is beneficial as long as it's in moderation. Children who are constipated, don't eat many whole fruits, or don't drink milk for their calcium source can all benefit from a daily half cup of orange or other 100 percent juice. The food guide pyramid for children presented in chapter 1 suggests two servings of fruit per day. These servings include, but are not limited to, one medium apple or banana, a half cup of chopped fruit, or one-third cup of 100 percent fruit juice.

Edible Energy

Protein plays an important role in the diet of a 4- to 6-year-old. Muscular development during these years requires a higher amount of essential amino acids found in quality protein sources. Complete protein foods such as milk, eggs, and meat are good choices for adequate intake of protein. As activity levels increase, so should caloric intake. Younger kids still need fewer calories per day compared with older kids and adults, so it's not a matter of eating more; it's a matter of eating well.

Easy Mixing

To help mix the oil that rises to the top of the jar of unhydrogenated peanut butter, store the jar upside down. That way, the oil rises to the bottom of the jar. Be sure to screw the top on tightly when you turn it upside down.

Typically 4- to 6-year-olds require about 30 calories per pound of body weight. This amount of energy is used to meet requirements for their growing bones and brains. To aid in more restful sleep, their bodies need to repair and rejuvenate, as well as receive enough energy to keep them playing nonstop. Growing kids need energy-dense foods, such as peanut butter, milk, and cheese as well as lower-energy foods, such as legumes and vegetables. Provide a balance of both types of foods at each meal. Sample meal plans and recipes can be found in chapters 9–12. The following table shows the suggested amount of daily nutrients for this age:

Nutrient Requirements per Day

Calories	1,600
Protein	31 grams
Fat	20 grams
Calcium	600 milligrams
Iron	10 milligrams
Vitamin A	500 micrograms
Vitamin C	45 milligrams
Vitamin D	5 milligrams

Good early care experiences expand your child's capacity to learn. Sometimes we worry whether we've done enough to give our kids a great start. Don't worry—you may already be doing many of the things that are best for your child. You can be more intentional about nurturing his brain development without fancy toys, software, or special equipment. Early childhood experiences exert an exciting impact and can physically determine how the brain is wired. Take the time now to provide an enriched environment for your kids. Expose them to many different experiences, each with the power to build up the ability to learn. Over the course of a week, try to incorporate the following exercises that promote connections between mind and body. These mental calisthenics can go a long way to improve brain function by preparing it to accept learning opportunities more easily.

Odd Man Out

At this age, kids are beginning to see the natural incongruities of life. They can categorize and group things by common elements. Gather together objects that have at least one element in common, but include one thing that is completely different with no common element. Ask your child, "Which one doesn't belong?" In the beginning, make it obvious. For example, a red block, a red apple, a red sock, a red bow, and a blue ball. Extend the game by asking your child what makes the block, the apple, the sock, and the bow the same.

What's Next?

Prediction is one of the cognitive skills that begin to develop between ages 4 and 6. Up until this point, kids may understand the words spoken to them but not necessarily the meaning behind them. If you tell your son or daughter not to pull the cat's tail because the cat won't like it, they may understand what you said but not why you said it. They don't yet have an experience that tells them the cat will retaliate! Practice prediction with children by observing common situations and ask them what may happen next. For example, if you are at the playground and you see a child kicking a ball too close to the street, ask your child, "Do you see that boy kicking the ball right next to the road? What could happen if he kicks it too hard?" Prediction helps develop the idea of consequences, both natural and imposed.

Making Faces

Kids' emotions at this age are becoming more and more adultlike. They experience the gamut! It still may be difficult for them to identify what they're feeling and be able to communicate those feelings to us. We all know how annoying it is when children pout. Often they're not even aware they're making a face. How many different emotions can they make faces for on demand? Write a set of emotions on slips of paper or index cards: happy, sad, mad, confused, frustrated, disappointed, and so forth. Put the emotions in a bag, have your child pick one out at random, and then make a face that goes with that emotion. Let the child give you the card so that you make a face, too. This will help you know what emotions your child can identify and which she can't. Connect the name of the emotion to the face and also a situation in which she might feel that emotion.

Shake, Rattle, and Roll

A sense of rhythm develops at this stage. Although some kids' sense of rhythm may be more or less developed at this age, all kids can benefit from "rhythm therapy." With or without musical accompaniment, clapping in time is a great rhythm producer. You may have played "Clap Hands" with your baby years ago, but now teach him how to clap to a song he knows. Have your child clap to mimic a rhythm you clap first. Then have your child come up with a rhythm for you to copy. Look for new ways to create rhythm using sticks, blocks, one key on the piano, or the tapping of his own feet.

What's That Smell?

Sensory learning helps us all create new connections. The sense of smell is one of the strongest connectors. There are pleasant smells and not so pleasant smells. You can formally set up a "smelling session" with your child by having her close her eyes while you place certain odors under her nose for identification. Consider using scented candles that give off a particular flower or flavor scent. Scratch-and-sniff books are available, too, for this very purpose. You can also just take advantage of the smells you come into contact with on a daily basis. Once you yourself sense a smell, stop and ask your child to close her eyes and guess what it is. For example, if you are outside on a cold winter's night and catch the smell of a fire in someone's fireplace, stop right in your tracks and say, "Close your eyes and smell the air. What do you smell?" If your child has trouble identifying the scent, tell her what it is. One way or the other she's made a new connection.

Drawing inside Your Mind

This exercise from Mark Singleton's book *Yoga for You and Your Child* has a calming, focusing effect and helps children develop their visual memory, which is important to their success in school. Sit down with your child in a quiet place, and have him close his eyes and relax. Ask your child to try to see a big piece of white paper inside his head. Tell him that he is going to imagine drawing some shapes on the paper in his mind. Then give your child some simple instructions about how to draw a basic shape or pattern. You might say, "First try to see yourself drawing a big circle. Inside the circle draw a square. Inside the square draw a triangle. Make sure none of the shapes touch each other." Pause between each direction, making sure your child is ready for the next. Finally, ask your child to open his eyes, give him a pencil and a piece of white paper, and ask him to really draw the shape or pattern he just visualized.

Chapter 5

7- TO 10-year-OLDS

A crust eaten in peace is better than
a banquet partaken in anxiety.
aesop

The playground was littered with kids. Janice sat on a nearby bench enjoying the scene in front of her like a well-rehearsed play. Jonathan found a friend on the climbing toy today. Thank goodness! He never wanted to stay long if he thought no one would play with him. Maybe today Janice could finish a conversation with Diane. Maybe 6-month-old Jessica would take her nap in the stroller today. Maybe Janice herself could enjoy an afternoon at the park. After all, she was set with everything they could possibly need. She had the first aid kit, extra diapers, Jessica's bottle, and a variety of snacks packed neatly into individual baggies for Jonathan.

Jonathan climbed to the top of the mass of twisted metal and tubing and stood on top of it. "Oh, no," Janice thought.

She leapt to her feet, jostling Jessica awake. Janice grabbed one of the snack baggies and stood directly underneath Jonathan at the climbing toy.

"Hey, how about something to eat?" she pleaded.

"Not hungry," Jonathan said and continued to walk as if on a tightrope.

"But it's your favorite—sour gummy worms," Janice said while waving the rainbow of wiggly candy worms at him.

Seconds later Jonathan sat quietly munching his worms on the bench next to Janice. Jessica had fallen back to sleep. Janice closed her eyes relieved to have avoided the verbal collision that was sure to follow had Jonathan remained on top of the climbing toy.

She knew he was more capable than years ago, but Jonathan's desire to be daring made Janice nervous. Would he grow into a careless daredevil in his teens? Janice knew that bribing him with sweets wasn't the best way to keep him safe, but sometimes it was the only thing that worked. She relaxed into her now-sleeping baby and whispered, "Stay just the way you are." Janice was in no hurry for this little one to be up and walking.

WHaT TO expeCT now

Kids at 7 to 10 years old are curious and like to learn. They read more fluently and absorb information more quickly—from understanding the rules of baseball to reading the food labels on the back of cartons. They're more aware of themselves and others. They can work independently but still need direction. They also work and play in groups but still need supervision. They are active, physically and intellectually. They enjoy team sports as well as solitary activities like reading or drawing. Around 8 years old, they become very social and really enjoy their friends.

The differences between boys and girls are more distinct now. Girls develop more quickly than boys, and you can see the changes coming on the outside. The girls are heavier and taller than many of the boys of the same age. Boys' changes are less noticeable for the next few years.

School gets more complicated for them now. According to teachers, third grade (at around age 9) is where the rubber meets the road. Kids with learning difficulties or differences are easily identified and offered special programming to meet their learning needs. During these intermediate elementary years, kids apply the basic skills they gained in kindergarten and first and second grades. Homework demands grow, and tests of all kinds are a regular part of the school year. Their minds are still quite flexible and open to new ideas, but at the close of this stage, the brain begins to wipe out the connections that haven't been used, making it harder to develop social, emotional, and intellectual skills. So as school gets more and more difficult, it's more and more important that we do everything we can to enable them as learners—and that includes their nutrition.

Sleep Tight

It's Monday at 6:00 A.M. and time to get your son up for school.

"I'm too tired. Let me sleep!" he yells.

"I know you're tired, but today is a school day and we all need to start moving," you say as pleasantly as possible.

"I don't want to go to school!" he whines and pulls the covers back over his head.

"You have to. Now get up!" you finally yell.

He does get up, but in a bad mood, and he won't eat breakfast. Then he's off to school, upset and hungry. What a way to start the day!

Sound familiar? We can all be tired, but if it gets in the way of our responsibilities, then it's a problem. Without adequate rest and nutrition, kids become handicapped learners at school. Disrupted or inconsistent sleep patterns make it difficult for any of us to function at our best. Bodies and minds function better with routine. Make sure your child goes to bed at the same time every night and gets up at the same time every morning. You determine your child's sleep habits, not your child.

School-aged kids require less sleep than babies or toddlers, but they still need about 10 hours per day. Your child's age, activity level, and health status strongly influence the amount of required sleep. Bedtime

---

Snooze Foods

- Dairy products: cottage cheese, cheese, milk
- Soy products: soy milk, tofu, soybean nuts
- Seafood
- Meats
- Poultry
- Beans
- Rice
- Hummus
- Hazelnuts, peanuts
- Sesame seeds, sunflower seeds
- Lentils
- Whole grains

rituals are still crucial at these ages. They can go to bed later as long as you figure in those 10 hours. Common fears such as fear of the dark, strange noises, intruders, or stress can disrupt your child's sleep. Some may even still have nightmares or night terrors. Be aware that what goes into your child before bedtime affects how well she sleeps. What she watches or reads, eats or drinks reduces or induces sleep. Kids at this age are not yet able to make these choices on their own; they need your guidance.

Sleep Inducers

Plan a healthy and calming evening snack after dinner if your child has difficulty falling asleep. Good choices for a bedtime snack are dairy products like milk, cheese, and eggs. Some other sleep-inducing foods are sesame seeds, hummus (a ground garbanzo bean dip), and brown rice. Mix any of these foods, and you'll have a snack that will get your child snoozing.

Try to avoid sugary desserts and caffeine-containing treats late in the day. Eating ice cream or a chocolate brownie soon before bed increases our energy when what we need is rest. Our bodies need to "reset" or come back to normal levels before lying down for the evening instead of gearing up for action.

Drink a glass of water before bed and keep one at the bedside for sips during the night (if awakened). It only takes 8 ounces of water in the evening to help the body's digestion run smoothly. Our body breaks up food from the day, little by little throughout the course of the night. Acting like a filter, water helps rid the body of waste and restore energy for the next day. Good mornings depend on good nights.

Food among Friends

Children in the intermediate grades of elementary school (third through fifth) transform from students who depend completely on their teachers to students who think and act independently. They are more able to sit still for longer periods of time, use language almost as fluently as adults, and have a great interest in competitive sports. They are also more apt to become distracted by their friends at school. Their self-control is challenged every day. They are tempted in how to behave, how to talk to adults, how to treat others, and even how and what to eat.

What your child eats depends on what you pack for lunch. Just because you pack it doesn't mean he eats it. Lunch trading and sharing are frequent activities in late elementary. A kid may want a certain snack in his lunch just because that's what his best friend brings. Usually he wants the same sugary snack and not the fruit a friend brings. He may feel pressure from friends to choose soda instead of milk.

School-Savvy Snacks

During these years, snack times of kindergarten and primary grades have been replaced with more academics. Some schools have read the research and provide "brain breaks" of nutritious snacks if they are provided by parents, but that is a teacher-by-teacher decision and is dependent on the choice of snack a parent provides for a class of 20 students. Most parents reach for a couple boxes of individually wrapped snack cakes for convenience when it is their turn to provide the class snack. It is just as easy to grab a bag of apples and individual cheese sticks to pass out at school. When it is your turn to feed the class, try checking out the outer aisles of the grocery store first. The high-sugar, prepackaged foods lie in the center aisles. Walk around the perimeter of a store first. You'll be surprised how easy it is to fill your cart with fresh, healthy foods. In chapter 12 we give many snack suggestions for countering the morning slump and the afternoon brain drain.

Where's the Water?

Most kids don't even drink water while at school, unless you send them with a bottle of water (if their school allows it). Water fountains may be broken, dispense warm water, or smell and harbor germs. Kids often avoid them. Water is an important part of our diet. It helps rid the body of waste and moves nutrients to where they're needed. All of our body functions work better when we have enough water in our tanks. Kids need to drink at least eight glasses a day of water. Most kids need more than the minimum, considering their naturally high activity levels. On average we lose a pint of water through our skin in the form of sweat each day. Replacing lost fluids regularly is important to our overall health.

What do you do if your kid doesn't like water—and he'd much rather drink fruit punch? This makes it more challenging to get in those eight glasses a day. First try adding a little flavor to water by dropping in a few ice cubes made from all natural fruit juices, frozen ahead of time. The added flavor might make it more appealing to him. Grocery stores now carry flavored water in all different flavors, from lemon to black cherry. Or, water down their favorite juice by adding $\frac{1}{2}$ cup of water to it—you'll increase their water intake and reduce the amount of sugar they take in from one glass of juice. As the weather turns cold, offer warm broth-type soups and baked potatoes for added water intake. During the summer, keep on hand plenty of fresh fruits and raw veggies. They all contain water that your child's body will use.

Brainy Breakfast

Often our kids go off to school without an adequate breakfast because we haven't built in the time they need to be hungry or the time we need to prepare it. Starting school without anything in your stomach is a recipe for disaster. If waking yourself or your child up earlier to ensure a quick breakfast is not a possibility, make sure she at least eats a snack the size of her fist that includes a protein and carbohydrate. A tablespoon of peanut butter mixed into a cup of yogurt or a pear and a cup of milk are both quick and easy choices for breakfast.

Children need the adequate nutrition to sustain their energy level and attentiveness throughout the day. And it's up to us to make sure they get it. Breakfast is the most important meal of the day for a reason. Our bodies are really in a state of fasting throughout the night. Brain function is minimal for survival, and the body is at rest. Once awake, stimuli bombard our brains, and we expect our bodies to do what we tell them to do. Without the necessary fuel, our minds are mush, and our bodies respond more like zombies. Make sure your child eats a balanced breakfast that provides the mental focus needed to start the day off right. Avoid sugar-laden cereals, and serve up a nutrient-dense breakfast instead. Chapters 9 to 12 include more detailed information about food choices, recipes, and meal plans.

Snack Attack

The competitive spirit begins to surface during these ages. If you want to give your child the edge, consider his nutritional needs. If he plays sports after school and on the weekends, he uses a greater amount of calories per day for energy. You can meet the extra demands on his body through nutrition so he gains stamina and continues to grow at a normal rate. Send him with a healthy after-school snack to eat to pump up his energy level before practice. If you don't provide this snack for energy, he might choose a soda or candy bar for a quick boost instead. Have available quick and healthy small meals or snacks, such as fruit, precut veggies, or yogurt. This helps ensure that he is getting the right balance of nutrients for his active and growing body.

Encouraging healthy snacking is a good way to add quality foods to your child's day. When you allow your child to have a snack, make sure it is not too close to a mealtime. You don't want to waste your carefully prepared dinner on an already-full belly. Snacking provides children with the energy to continue through the day on an even level. Bananas, dried fruits, melons, yogurts, or low-fat cream cheese spread with crackers are some examples of healthful snacks. Snacking should be used to help us get from one part of the day to the next. Snacks help us avoid the pitfalls of low energy between typical mealtimes. Many suggestions of brain booster foods and healthy meal plans appear in chapter 12 and appendix B, respectively.

The Turtle and the Hare

Children come in all shapes and sizes. Even within one family, there can be children of different body types and metabolism. *Metabolism* is the process of converting the food we eat into energy. A child with a fast metabolism can eat a large amount of food and not gain weight, whereas a child with a slower metabolism can continue to gain weight even when consuming fewer calories daily. As long as both children are selecting nutrient-dense foods to eat and are both physically active each day, there should be little concern of obesity or growth problems. We need to remember that we all have different bone structures and amounts of muscle mass versus fat weight. Size differences affect the efficiency of our metabolism.

A Satisfying Self-Image

Children need to be reminded that they are special and unique in every way, including their body type. When girls at this age start to worry about diet, weight, or size, it's a red flag to get involved. Girls are especially vulnerable at this age. Their bodies are beginning to change, and they are not sure if they like the change. Young girls look outward to find acceptance. They read magazines that equate beauty with ultra-thin models. They focus on outside beauty, and the number on the scale becomes their measure of self-worth.

We can reassure our daughters about their individuality and the importance of health through nutrition, not trends. Remind them that food is our energy lifeline and not an enemy to our self-esteem. This message should be clear and consistent through our own actions and words. If they see us obsess about our weight and appearance, they will pick up on that even if we're telling them something completely different.

Jumps and Jiggles

Encourage an active lifestyle for your kids and join them when they jump and jiggle. Choose family activities that encourage movement and fitness.

Mood and Food

Mixing food types, such as carbohydrates and a protein-rich food, cut fruit with nuts, or wheat crackers and cheese, allows for a balanced snack. Children need the balance from foods to help keep their blood sugar levels on an even keel. Children's mood and energy levels depend on their blood sugar levels. An inconsistent or inadequate amount of combined nutrients wreaks havoc on hormones, which are the core of behavioral responses. Balance sugar throughout the day—your child's teacher will thank you.

The Diabetes Dilemma

Children with diabetes need to regulate their blood sugar levels with the help of the hormone insulin. Their body no longer produces enough insulin on its own to regulate the highs and lows of blood sugar. These swings in blood sugar can cause a wide range of unwanted behavior and emotions in children, from hyperactivity and an inability to concentrate to depression and sleepiness.

The focus of treatment for diabetes in children is to control their blood sugar levels within a safe range. Testing blood sugar several times a day or whenever your child has symptoms of high or low blood sugar is the first step in treatment. The second step is taking insulin injections as prescribed by your doctor. Third, monitor your child's daily diet and exercise routine. You can do this by spreading out your child's consumption of carbs throughout the day to stop blood sugar spikes. Kids need snacks throughout the day that have a balance between protein and carbohydrates to steady their blood sugar. Good examples are cheese sticks with a handful of nuts, wheat crackers topped with cream cheese or peanut butter (or both), and yogurt mixed with berries or granola.

After a healthy snack, don't forget to get your kids moving. Aim for exercise and physical play for at least 60 minutes most days of the week. For more information on childhood diabetes, contact the Juvenile Diabetes Research Foundation at www.jdrf.org.

Satisfy Your Carbs

Beginning a meal with a complex carbohydrate food and a protein, such as whole wheat pasta and low-fat cheese, and eating it slowly will lessen your craving for fats during the rest of the meal. You will start to feel full and won't want as much high-fat food.

The TV Guide

Television strongly influences kids' eating habits at this age, and food manufacturers know that. That's why they gear their commercials to kids. Sit down in the afternoon and watch television *with* your kids. Then count how many commercials advertise "kid" foods (meals, cereals, snacks, drinks, etc.). You'll be amazed! "Kid" foods are usually higher in sugar and less nutritious. The ads on TV make "junk" food appealing to kids with their colorful packaging and cartoon character promoters, so beware when you take your kids with you to the grocery store. If you're not careful, the TV becomes your child's guide to food instead of you.

Mixed Messages

Don't confuse your kids. Leave junk food on the shelf at the supermarket, not in your pantry! And give treats other than food as rewards to kids. Giving candy to kids as a reward or a treat confuses children when they are learning nutritional values of foods. "How can a treat not give me nutrition?" they wonder.

Overcoming Obesity

Childhood obesity is growing rapidly in the United States. Obesity means a person having a body fat percentage higher than 30 percent. Body fat in children increases for a number of reasons. Poor nutritional choices, family history, and physical inactivity are all factors

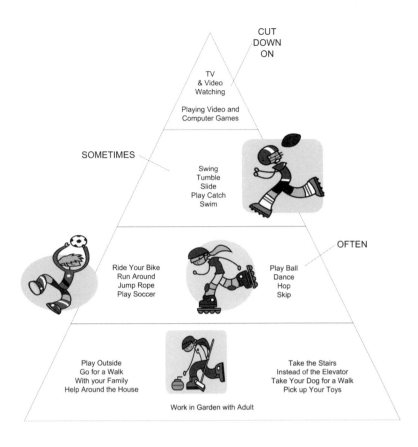

CUT
DOWN
ON

TV
& Video
Watching

Playing Video and
Computer Games

SOMETIMES

Swing
Tumble
Slide
Play Catch
Swim

OFTEN

Ride Your Bike
Run Around
Jump Rope
Play Soccer

Play Ball
Dance
Hop
Skip

Play Outside
Go for a Walk
With your Family
Help Around the House

Take the Stairs
Instead of the Elevator
Take Your Dog for a Walk
Pick up Your Toys

Work in Garden with Adult

that help tip the scales. Obesity in childhood can lead to the development of a host of medical problems, including hypertension and respiratory infections now and later in life. You are probably thinking, "Just don't feed your kids so much" or "That child must eat *a lot* to be that big at his age." However, the amount of caloric intake in a child's diet has not significantly increased, but a decrease in quality food consumption, such as fruits and vegetables, is as much as 25 percent among school-age children. One-quarter of American children consume vegetables from potatoes in the form of French fries and chips. Their "choice" of vegetable is popular, but not nutritious.

The decline of physical activity also contributes to the increase in childhood obesity. As a nation we exercise too little and indulge in low-quality foods too often. Television is one of the biggest blocks children have to getting to exercise. They spend more time on the virtual playing fields of their computer games than outside in their own yards or at a park. Encourage your child to put down the controller and head outside for some hiking, jump roping, rollerblading, and so forth. Our kids need to eat more fresh fruits and veggies on a daily basis, and they need to get moving. It is our job to help this happen by providing a good example of eating and activity; keeping healthy snacks available on a regular basis and including them at every meal; insisting on physical activity, at least an hour a day, for your kids. You can go for walks or exploring hikes together as a family or play a game of Marco Polo together in the pool. Do it as a family or encourage sport activities for your kids to join, but just do it!

Better Butter

As a healthier alternative to butter, mix butter with canola oil. Put two sticks of butter into a blender with one cup canola oil. Blend until smooth. Drop in 1 tablespoon of lecithin (found in health stores). Store in the refrigerator in a covered container.

Edible Energy

Seven- to 10-year-olds need approximately 1,600–2,400 calories a day. At most ages boys require more calories than girls because of their larger bone and muscle structure. But appetites can vary from child to child and even from day to day. For example, a child doing homework all afternoon may have fewer caloric needs than one who is at soccer practice after school. The following table provides nutritional amounts needed daily for a 7- to 10-year-old:

Vitamin and Mineral Requirements Daily

Calcium	800–1,200 milligrams
Iron	10 milligrams
Vitamin A	700 micrograms
Vitamin C	45 milligrams
Vitamin D	5 micrograms

THE ELEMENTARY BRAIN

At this point in their development, kids lose more brain connections (synapses) than they make. At age 8 months, an infant may have 1,000 trillion synapses; but by age 10, the number of synapses decreases to about 500 trillion. We can help increase the number of synapses by helping our child make new connections. The brain actually builds itself if we provide it with the right tools. Each sensory experience—what a child sees, hears, touches, tastes, and smells—creates connections between brain cells. Repeated experiences solidify these connections and promote learning and understanding. Over the course of a week, try to incorporate the following exercises to promote connections between mind and body. Aligned to an effective work-out routine, these mental calisthenics can go a long way to improve brain function by preparing it to accept learning opportunities more easily.

Eye Spy

This is a variation on the game we've all played while riding in the car. This time tie in things your children may currently be learning in school. "Eye spy *la roja boca*," or "Eye spy a freckled femur," or "Eye spy a cream-colored canine" each represent something children may be learning in school and force their minds to think past the expected.

The Real Deal

Memory is improved when the memory is meaningful. Look for ways to make meaningful connections with your children about something they've read, watched on television, seen on the playground, or heard in school. Even reading a fairy tale can be relevant to your child's everyday life. Consider the tale of Little Red Riding Hood. Can your child relate to Red Riding Hood's desire to see her grandmother? Does she remember a time when she might have gone a different way than you told her to? If it's relevant, they'll remember it!

Starts With

The ability to generate many ideas with ease shows fluent thinking. When you find yourselves waiting, whether you're in the car, in the doctor's office, or standing in line somewhere, play this word game with your children. "Let's think of movies that start with the letter *L*" or "Let's think of foods that start with *S*." Take turns naming something that starts with that letter. If the answer is a two- or three-word answer, each word must start with that letter as well. This game is difficult for some kids and adults in the beginning, but over time you are able to think of answers more quickly and for longer periods of time.

Novel Idea

Encourage your child to engage in an activity that is new to him. If his favorite type of book is mystery, encourage him to read a biography. If her favorite sport is soccer, encourage her to try gymnastics. There is no guarantee that children will excel in these new activities, but the point is that they will create new connections and strengthen their synapses.

Do You Hear What I Hear?

Helping our kids focus on a particular sense increases their ability to retain information. Let's focus on *hearing*. Sit outside and have everyone close their eyes and remain perfectly still. Ask them to focus on all the different sounds they may hear. They may hear traffic noises, leaves rustling, birds singing, a dog barking, or their own breathing.

Imagine

Visualization as a relaxation technique slows the heart rate and relaxes the muscles. It also can clear the mind and help reduce stress. Our kids are overscheduled with very little time to just relax. Help them practice to be still as a way to allow their minds to renew and their bodies to recharge. Lie on the soft grass outside, in your own bed, or even on the floor of your comfy living room and close your eyes. Allow your arms to fall to your sides and your feet to fall open. This is the yoga pose called the corpse pose (but you don't have to tell them that!). Allow each part of your body to soften from your face down to your toes, part by part. Encourage your child to let their thoughts float away like clouds. Relax completely for at least 5 minutes this way.

Chapter 6

11- TO 14-year-OLDS

The dinner table is the center for the teaching
and practicing not just of table manners but of
conversation, consideration, tolerance, family feeling,
and just about all the other accomplishments
of polite society except the minuet.
JUDITH MARTIN (MISS MANNERS)

Susan unpacked her car of the cooler full of orange slices and granola bars, grabbed her 6-year-old by the hand, and headed toward the baseball fields. The team mother shouldn't be late for the game, but somehow Susan always was. She delivered the snacks to the coach and scanned the outfield for John. There he was in right field. She was disappointed for him. He had really hoped the coach would give him a chance at the infield this game. Susan pressed her face against the chain link fence trying to catch her son's eye. He didn't see her, or he wouldn't look at her—it was hard to tell these days.

Six-year-old Jessie pulled on Susan's coat sleeve. "Can I go to the playground now?" she asked.

"Not yet," Susan said. "I need to watch your brother play his game."

"But I want to play, too. Can't I go by myself?"

Susan knew this would be one long game if Jessie continued to bug her about going to play. But she'd never missed one of John's games, and she wasn't sure how it would go over if she just disappeared to the other side of the park. What if John looked for her and didn't see her watching him? Their relationship was tenuous as it was. She didn't want to make things worse.

"Please, Mommy," Jessie whined. "I can go by myself. Please."

There was no way Susan would let Jessie go to the playground on her own. She was still too young, and Susan's fear of her being snatched overruled her big-eyed, blonde sweetheart.

At the end of the third inning, the outfield trotted into the dugout. Susan stuck her head in and called John. He didn't respond. She called again.

John came to the edge of the dugout and said, "Mooommmm, what?"

There was that tone again. The one that said, "You're embarrassing me, Mom. Leave me alone!"

"I'm going to take your sister to the playground until the game is over," she said.

"Fine," John said.

"Is that OK with you? That I won't see the rest of your game?"

"Whatever," John said. He already started walking back to the bench.

As Susan headed for the playground with Jessie running ahead, she didn't know whether to be happy that John didn't seem to always need her right there anymore or to be sad that her little boy was disappearing.

WHAT TO EXPECT NOW

Eleven- to 14-year-olds grow on every level, ranging from cantankerous to calm and back again. Energy levels continue to increase right along with appetite levels. They need a lot of energy but less sleep. Physically we see rapid height and weight growth. Hormones wreak havoc on both girls and boys. They have mixed emotions about themselves and everyone around them. Moodiness and "attitude issues" plague the preteen. Daily challenges like getting to class on time, finding lockers, and keeping up with the school workload are enough to make your child lock herself in her room and say, "Leave me alone!" Mood swings are common and easily affected by inside and outside pressures. As your preteen works toward independence, she has more responsibilities (which she likes) and less free time (which she hates). She wants to be independent, but she's realizing, probably for the first time, that there's a price to pay.

Academically, some students who traditionally did well in school experience failure or ambivalence toward learning at around age 12. As they look for self-definition, they use complaints and criticism to gain attention from others. Being confrontational seems to be their goal at this age. Since these years are filled with turbulence and confusion, it's a great time for parents to be supportive and validate their child's emotions and feelings. Try to enjoy the energy of your child at this age. They're no longer too young or too small to do most things, and you can spend more time as a family in shared activities like games, sports, travel, and events you are all interested in.

Jack and the Beanstalk

How tall will my daughter be?

Mom, everyone is bigger than me. When will I grow?

I think my son is not tall enough for sports. When will he be the right size?

These questions are common, but their answers are complex and depend on many variables. Height and weight charts, body mass index (BMI) calculations, and genetics give us a peak into future height expectations of boys. Don't worry about children's height at this age unless they don't grow taller for 6 months to 1 year.

Adolescence is a time of growth spurts. Boys will add on lots of height and weight at this time. They will also keep growing until they're about 23 but will reach 90 percent of their adult height by the age of 18. Girls' growth spurt is younger and usually peaks at around age 15.

Fitting in Is Hard to Do

"Mom, Susie just got the coolest pair of jeans. Can I get some like hers?" asked Shelly.

"Sure. How about these?" said Mom.

"No, Mom. They're more like these!" Shelly held up a pair of straight, too-small-looking pants.

"Honey, I don't think those are appropriate for school or your size. Let's find another style," said Mom.

"But Mom! This is the best pair. I want these. Everyone has them!"

"Shelly, we're not getting jeans that are too tight for you! Maybe, after you lose a few pounds. How about we try the next size up?"

"They are supposed to fit that way, Mom! You don't understand."

"I don't want you wearing jeans that you can't sit down in. And that's final!"

"You're not fair!" cried Shelly.

By age 11, girls become aware of their appearance and want to "fit in" with the crowd. The added pounds and hormones to a girl's body make "fitting in" more difficult by raising her level of frustration and self-doubt. This new focus causes many girls to diet when their bodies really need more fuel, not less fuel. Some parents even encourage their daughters to diet or "watch" their eating. This sends mixed messages to girls as they try to understand which is better, being healthy or being thin.

The fact is that pubescent girls who go on restrictive diets to lose weight or fit into a pair of jeans are setting themselves up for future health problems. Imagine if a carpenter cut the wood supply list short while building a house—it would make for a weak model. It might still "look good" from the outside, but that house couldn't withstand nature's fury. Girls are "building" themselves now for the future. Help your daughter realize the importance of her health over hip-hugger jeans.

Support your daughter with positive feedback. Start by asking her what sports or activities she enjoys, and join her doing some of them. Include her when you plan weekly meals and grocery lists. Encourage her to help make dinner once a week. Vary the supply of fruits and vegetables, and make sure grains and dairy are always available in your home. Keep in mind that if you don't buy it or bake it, she (and you) will not have a difficult time avoiding junk food. By your own example, you can give your daughter the message that a healthy and physically strong body is what builds self-esteem.

Puberty's Promise

Puberty is all about change. The body is retooling for adult roles and responsibilities. Puberty brings on growth spurts and menstruation in girls, beginning around 11 years old. Right now girls need more calories and more iron in their diets. The amount of iron lost during menstruation needs to be replaced through what they eat or with an iron supplement; otherwise, you'll notice an increase in fatigue and mood-iness in your "little" girl.

As curves and added body fat begin to develop, so does a girl's body awareness. She should grow into her weight after puberty, which ends at around age 15.

Puberty for boys starts around age 12 and ends at around age 17. The increase of hormones flooding their bodies causes a noticeable change in their appearance. Added muscular mass in boys demands a higher need for protein and calories. Sexual development and voice changes also happen now. Emotionally they experience new and confusing feelings. Their hormones are soaring while their energy levels plummet. However, all changes require energy: physical and emotional. They need more protein and calories to meet their new energy needs. Refer to the table later in this chapter for the proper amount of nutrients required.

Leaner Calories

You are less likely to gain fat weight while eating complex carbohydrates than you are from the same number of calories from fat. Most people burn a higher proportion of the calories from carbohydrates during the digestion process than they do from the same amount of fat.

Aggravating Acne

Acne is almost a universal affliction for adolescents. Even one or two pimples can cause much worrying in front of a mirror. A face full of acne can result in permanent scarring of the skin and psyche. Acne cannot be cured, but it can be treated with topical medications as well as a change in diet.

It is important to first mention that diet in itself does not cause acne, but a diet high in sugar and fat and low in zinc and vitamin A will make matters worse. A diet with at least five servings a day of fruits and veggies helps support the immune system and decreases skin inflammations. The best way to get zinc and vitamin A is to eat more fresh fruits and vegetables. Dark green veggies (spinach) contain higher amounts of zinc; orange/red veggies or fruits (carrots or apples) for vitamin A are great examples. If we eat a rainbow of colorful fresh veggies and fruits over the course of a week, we boost our immune system and keep sickness at bay.

Even though the cause of acne has not been definitively determined, heredity does play a role. If you had acne, there is a good chance your child will, too. During adolescence, bodies begin to produce an increased amount of male hormones called *androgens*. Girls also produce these hormones, but only one-tenth as much. The exact role hormones play in the development of acne is not known.

A number of other factors can cause, contribute, or trigger the development of acne besides heredity and puberty:

- Some drugs, including certain hormones, epilepsy drugs, and antituberculosis medicines
- Exposure to industrial oils and chemicals, such as PCBs
- Certain types of bacteria, such as corynebacterium
- Stress and strong emotions, such as guilt, anxiety, and fear
- The onset of menstruation in girls each month
- Birth control pills
- Some oily cosmetics and shampoos

Certain foods, such as chocolate, nuts, cola drinks, French fries, potato chips, and other fatty or junk foods may make acne worse and exacerbate the condition, but not cause it directly.

The PB&J Myth

"Mom, I want peanut butter and jelly for lunch tomorrow."

"Honey, why don't you try a new sandwich?"

"But I only like PB&J!"

How can we get our kids to branch out and try new foods? When it comes to cold lunches, some get fixated on one type of sandwich. How do we get them to eat a balanced meal when they only eat peanut butter and jelly? Typically kids like white bread spread with peanut butter and a high-sugar jelly. Many parents are happy to see their kids eating a sandwich and believe that they're getting a little protein from the peanut butter. Truth be told, peanut butter is an incomplete protein that doesn't supply all the amino acids on its own. The white bread has been bleached and stripped of most natural fiber and vitamins. Add to the mix a tablespoon of sugar, the main ingredient of most jellies, and you've given your kid a high-sugar, low-nutrient sandwich that will not fill her belly for very long before she gets tired and cranky from the inevitable sugar crash.

A balanced nutritious lunch comes in all shapes and sizes. Lunch doesn't have to equal a sandwich. Most of us get stuck between two slices of bread. Try adding variety to the type of lunches your kids eat.

If he likes peanut butter, serve it on a whole grain slice of bread with sliced bananas on top. Peanut butter and apple wedges or celery sticks is another way to make a more complete protein snack. Wheat crackers stacked with sliced low-fat cheese, turkey diced with cut cucumbers, and yogurt with berries—voilà! You've got lunch.

Fiber for the Family

In addition to being a friend to aging bowels, fiber is also valuable for school-age children. It delays the absorption rate of sugars in the food to the bloodstream, consequently helping children behave and learn better, without the interruptions of hyperactivity from sugar highs.

Tummy Troubles

Stress plays a large role in the life of a preteen. Their physical and emotional development is booming. Puberty in itself causes stress inside and out. Children deal with stress in different ways. Physical activity helps relieve some of that stress. New problems can occur when children hold in their feelings. Stomachaches are a common way stress exacerbates itself and a red flag to you that something is wrong.

Joey wakes up every Monday with a stomachache. He complains of pain only in the morning and goes through the rest of his day fine. The doctor says he's probably constipated. Even after treating him for constipation, Joey still complains of stomach pain. Emotional stress at school or home may be contributing to Joey's upset stomach. Children at this age experience many changes beyond their own control. As they struggle toward independence, they either internalize their feelings or "act out" and get into trouble. Support them by practicing patience and understanding, and try not to overcriticize or demand a change in their feelings or behavior. Encourage some extracurricular activities.

Physical activity is a healthy way to "deal" with the many physical and emotional changes by building both muscle and a more positive self-image. Try to encourage your child to participate in a team sport or club. Yoga and karate are two activities that promote relaxation, a strong sense of self, and a mind—body balance that can all help reduce the stress in your child's life.

Eat Sweets on a Full Stomach

Downing a 12-ounce can of sugary soda on an empty stomach is more likely to trigger the insulin roller coaster and adrenaline rush than drinking that same soda with a meal. Save the sweets for an after-meal treat. A high-sugar breakfast is another roller-coaster starter. It sets up the school-age child for a midmorning crash.

An Athlete's Advantage

While being physically active is a positive thing, it puts greater demands on a still-growing body. If your child strives to be a top athlete or is training for an upcoming competition, be more mindful of her nutrition needs in order to give her a leg up and extra protection. The extra energy and time spent on these activities needs to be balanced with added rest and optimal nutrition. Without adequate rest and quality nutrition, illness and injuries happen more frequently.

Help your young athlete meet the extra demands on her body and heighten her performance level by making sure she gets the necessary added calories through frequent snacking. Especially include snacks high in carbohydrates and mixed with protein. Carbs such as bananas or spaghetti will provide extra energy, while proteins like cheese, peanut butter, or turkey meatballs will help build muscles.

Your child's body will also need lots and lots of water. Kids need to stay hydrated to avoid heat exhaustion or passing out on the field. Make sure your young athlete drinks water before, during, and after games and practices.

Unfortunately, some kids begin to experiment with stimulant drugs like caffeine and speed instead of food to raise their energy levels. The use of such drugs puts a strain on their immune system, and they are not hard to find, which makes them difficult to control. Caffeinated beverages fill the vending machines at school, and "uppers" are found in your local convenience store as drugs to keep you awake all night.

Make sure your young athlete eats breakfast before school and gets enough good food at lunch, and try sending him with fruit and bottled water in his backpack for after-school practices. This helps him get the energy boost he needs for practice *without* stopping by the soda machine or local corner market.

Fruit Snacks

Fruits that contain higher amounts of fructose relative to glucose and sucrose are the most blood sugar–friendly snacks. The primary sugar in pears and apples is fructose, which, combined with the high fiber content of these fruits, should produce steady sugar absorption, without the spikes of sugar highs and lows.

Couch Potatoes

Some children prefer playing electronic games to playing outside. Inside the "playroom" of many homes there is a television, a video game system, and a computer. These recreation choices don't promote interaction with other people and decrease the desire for physical activity. At an age when growth is high, inactivity from sitting in front of a television screen doesn't benefit a child's physical development. So what do we do when our kids only want to play electronic games?

The average child between the ages of 7 and 13 spends close to 4 hours each day watching television or playing electronic games. American children are becoming increasingly less active with each year of life. Parents can set an example and participate in physical activities like playing catch or riding bikes. Encourage regular physical activity now, and you help your child become physically active for a lifetime.

You can combat inactivity by limiting sedentary activities and encouraging physical ones. One guideline to follow is to limit sedentary time to no more than 1 hour at any given point in the day. Sedentary time includes computer games, television shows, and even reading. Encourage your teen to take a break from one of these activities after about an hour. Plan at least an hour a day of structured activity geared toward a specific skill. Practice batting swings, dribbling, kicking goals, or learning to jump rope. These physical activities can be done in 15-minute bouts or an hour at a time. Recreation activities for the mind and the body should be mixed and alternated throughout the day to develop a balance of mood and function in your teen. One way to help your kids find a balance is to suggest time limits. "After 40 minutes of video games, it's time to go outside." This will nudge them to transition from one activity to another.

The Dinner Delight

Even if every other meal during the day didn't go the way you planned, dinner at home can help balance the scales. Keep in mind that it may be the only meal that you have complete control over as a parent. Between school, work, and your child's extracurricular activities, there seems to be no time to sit together for a home-cooked meal, but with a little planning you can give your family what they need even if you're not all together at the table.

Slow cookers and crock pots make preparing nutritious and delicious meals a snap even for parents who both work outside the home. Refer to chapter 11 for many healthy suggestions for quick meals. Another book, *Once a Month Cooking* by Beth Lagerborg, suggests taking one day a month to cook and freeze nightly meals ahead of time. This is your chance to combat the skipped breakfast, the school cafeteria lunch, and the quick-pick candy bar on the way home. Include the missing nutrients during dinner, and you can be confident that your kids got what they needed.

The Seventh Grade Slump

For many kids, seventh grade is a part of middle school. It is a year of transition for learning and maturity. Parents and teachers of seventh graders wrestle daily with kids with major mood swings, little focus, and rare moments of common sense or organization. Even kids who did well in school until now may have difficulty. Suddenly their grades drop, and their interest in things they once enjoyed wanes. They have six or sometimes seven teachers with separate expectations, homework, projects, and activities. Kids who aren't naturally organized flounder and sometimes experience failure for the first time.

Maturity is measured by their ability to be responsible, but they are just learning what that means in their daily life. They may be quite capable in math, but since they forget to do their homework, they'll get poor grades. Support this transition by offering your child ways to get and stay organized. Monitor progress at school weekly, and conference with your child often. Help him to set goals and then give him the tools he needs to meet those goals. If he wants to be able to remember to do his homework, help him come up with a system using a planner or an assignment sheet. Partner with teachers for his success in these areas. This is definitely not the time to walk away or become less involved in his schooling. You may find yourself more involved than you like, but until he can manage his school life successfully on his own, it's your job.

Edible Energy

In order to reduce illnesses, stress, and fatigue from the demands of their busy lifestyle, preteens need to consume nutrient-rich foods as often as possible. Physical activity also needs to be balanced with the food they eat. Supply a diet with plenty of grain products, vegetables, and fruits. Moderate sugar intake and saturated fat, and choose foods that provide enough calcium and iron to meet their growing needs.

Three Sweet Beans

If you or your child is a sugar-sensitive person, try a three-bean salad. Kidney beans, chickpeas, and pinto beans all have low glycemic indexes. No sugar highs here, just good, steady nutrition.

Balanced nutrition and stable blood sugar levels can ease this transitional time. Eating low-nutrient and high-sugar foods will only add to preteens' ups and downs. Many kids eat on the run or skip meals, which decreases the balance of nutrient intake and increases the likelihood of moodiness and fatigue.

Adolescence is a hard time for children and their parents. Unbalanced nutrition complicates matters and causes more problems in the long run. The following table shows the amount of nutrients needed for a preteen:

Nutrient Requirements per Day

Calories	2,200–2,500
Protein	45 grams
Iron	15 milligrams
Zinc	12 milligrams
Calcium	1,300 milligrams
Vitamin A	50 milligrams
Vitamin C	1,000 micrograms
Vitamin D	10 IU

The preteen brain is beginning to process information in a completely different way. It moves from understanding life through concrete ideas to more abstract ideas. Kids at this age don't have to touch something to understand it. They can connect ideas like love, truth, justice, or loyalty through their experiences and conversations. They can take large leaps in logic at the end of this stage, and it's important to offer opportunities to process their experiences with logic. Focus on helping preteens think more critically about why they and others do what they do. Discuss what they see in the news, and talk about how it could impact their lives.

Over the course of a week, try to incorporate the following exercises that promote connection between mind and body. These mental calisthenics can go a long way to improve brain function by preparing it to accept learning opportunities more easily.

Walk It Off

A common complaint during this age is a poor attitude. Attitude can affect children's willingness to learn. Often they just need a change of scenery or change of position. Our teens and preteens sit more often than they do anything else. Let's warm them up by getting them moving.

Go for a brisk walk around the block with your child. Once or twice around is sufficient to get the blood flowing and to sweep away the cobwebs of an "I don't care" attitude. Make it an easy and relaxed time together—no talk of "should's" or "have to's" or "What's wrong with you?" When you return home, drink a full glass of water before sitting down to do anything that is school related.

Cross Crawls

Movements that focus on crossing the midline in the body and the brain are used to connect both sides, which can improve coordination of seeing, hearing, and touching and academic skills like spelling, writing, listening, and reading comprehension. These exercises can be found in Dennison and Dennison's book *Brain Gym*. Similar to walking in place, the child alternately moves one arm and its opposite leg and the other arm and its opposite leg. You can vary this exercise by having your child do it while sitting, with eyes closed, or to music.

What's It Good For?

Generating ideas is sometimes difficult without a purpose or goal in mind. Focused brainstorming can help the child who comes up with one idea and believes it is the only one possible. Have him consider a common object, such as sunglasses. Now ask him to come up with 12 different uses for sunglasses. This is asking him to think of things that sunglasses normally aren't used for. His first response may be "To block the glare of the sun." That's the expected answer. Push him to consider strange and more unexpected answers. Examples might include to hide a black eye, wear a disguise, use for cutting, look like a movie star, use as a mirror, hold back hair from face, protect eyes from dirt, and so forth.

Forced Relationships

Students at this age tend to get easily stumped when asked to come up with ideas—ideas for a story, ideas for a report, ideas for art class, or ideas for a science fair project. Once stumped, they stop right in their tracks. The following exercise will help them generate ideas in a more systematic way and avoid the "I don't know!" automatic response.

Many things exist today that combine two previously unrelated things into something new. Consider the clock radio, the PDA, and many other new technologies that combine multiple functions into something new. One way to envision new ideas is to use a forced relationships matrix.

List items or ideas on the left side and the same items or others listed across the top. In the box where each one meets, a new association has been made. Have your child try it for herself using foods and types of preparation. On the left side of the matrix, list foods your child likes. Across the top list ways in which different foods are prepared—baked, fried, broiled, and so on. Where the boxes meet, see if a new association has been made that looks appetizing. This is great for generating ideas for stories, new sports, board games, or experiments.

Touch and Go

Preteens and teens are very physical beings. They need opportunities to connect either touch or movement with what they learn. This exercise is a touch scavenger hunt. For example, say, "Go find and touch in order five things that are wood, four things that are plastic, three things that are fabric, two things that are metal, and one liquid item." You can vary this exercise by aligning it with something your child is currently learning: shapes for geometry, living things for biology, or even giving the instructions in a language they are studying.

What Happened Today?

Usually when you ask preteens or teens what they did today or what they did in school today, their answer is "Nothing." Bedtime is still a good time to recap the day's events and empty the mind to encourage a more restful sleep. Ask your child to close his eyes and relax. Tell him he is going to remember all the things that have happened to him today beginning with the present moment and working backward through the day until he gets to the morning when he was still lying in bed, just like a movie playing backward. Prompt him periodically if he gets stuck, but don't push too hard. Let him tell you as much detail as he wants. He may give up halfway through the exercise, which is normal. As he becomes more and more comfortable with visualization, he will reveal more and more.

Chapter 7

15- TO 18-YEAR-OLDS

If we could give every individual the right amount of
nourishment and exercise, not too little and not too much,
we would have found the safest way to health.

HIPPOCRATES

Sam wrestled his backpack out of the back of his parents' Suburban and headed toward the school. The familiar beep of a horn made him turn slightly back toward the car. His mom waved and smiled at him. Sam waved back with only his pinkie finger and then hustled into the building. Although he was glad his mom drove him to school so he wouldn't have to ride the bus, Sam wished she wouldn't make such a big deal out of it.

After school, Sam walked to the practice fields at a nearby park with the rest of the track team. He sat on the ground and quietly ate the snack his mom prepared. He wouldn't get home until well after dinner, so she sent him with enough fuel to get through the next 5 hours: an orange, a bologna sandwich, tortilla chips, soda, and two water bottles. He couldn't get through practice without those water bottles.

"Get rid of the soda," Coach K said.

"But it's my drink," Sam said.

"Not if you want to be on my team," said Coach. "No sugar, remember?"

Sam poured the soda into the nearby garbage can and then put the can in his backpack to recycle once he got home.

"What's in the sandwich?" asked Coach.

"Bologna," said Sam.

"Processed meat. Well, I'll let you get away with that today, but next time make sure your protein isn't processed," Coach said. He moved on to the next food victim sitting on the grass.

Great, Sam thought. Now I've got to tell Mom that Coach doesn't like the snacks she makes for me.

As a 1,600 runner, Sam had to make sure his body fat was low and his energy sources could sustain him at a steady pace for the mile run. No simple sugars, but a diet high in protein and complex carbs. Sam learned more about nutrition from running track than he did in health class! It was the edge he needed if he was going to hold his front-runner standing on the team.

WHAT TO EXPECT NOW

Adolescence is usually not an easy time for teens or parents. New challenges will test your patience, understanding, and parenting skills. By the age of 15, teens want control over more aspects of their life. Older teenagers are more self-assured and better able to resist peer pressure. Teens still need parents to set limits, even if they won't admit it. Base rules and privileges on your child's level of maturity, not chronological age. Some limits parents can employ affect curfews, driving privileges, and dating. Parents also need to insist on and model a healthy lifestyle, which includes adequate nutrition, physical activity, and frequent family mealtimes.

Teens frequently question and challenge school and parental rules. Intellectually, they are better able to solve problems and use organizational skills. Many teens successfully juggle school, outside activities, and work. But they are often so busy that eating right is last on their list of priorities. Although we want our teens to be independent thinkers and not follow the crowd, we still secretly want a measure of control. This is the time of helping kids accept responsibility for their own choices, even if those choices aren't always the best.

Eat Now, Think Later

Making food choices is just like making friends for teens. It's a decision they make for the immediate benefit, not for the long run. They sometimes choose friends out of convenience; they're on the same baseball team, or they have the same class schedule or have similar interests. Teens don't think about next year or when they graduate; they think about right now. Choosing foods is the same way. They eat what's convenient. They eat what their friends eat where their friends eat. It doesn't matter to *them* if they don't actually like much of what is offered in the school cafeteria, even though it matters to *you*. Your desire to still make sure your child eats right must be balanced by letting him make his own decisions. It's a definite balancing act, but well worth the effort.

Don't Skin the Iron

Leave the skin on the potatoes when making homemade fries. This way you'll get more nutrition into the French fry–loving picky eater. The potato skin is rich in nutrition and contains five times the amount of iron as the whole rest of the potato.

Weight Matters

Weight management and childhood obesity are central concerns of parents. At the other ends of the spectrum are teens who are undernourished, not due to poverty but to pressure. Although their current weight is normal, many girls feel pressured to be "ideally" thin like models and actresses in movies and magazines. An increasing number of girls between the ages of 12 and 18 suffer at least one bout with an eating disorder, such as anorexia nervosa, which causes people to severely limit their caloric intake in an effort to reach extreme thinness. Another common eating disorder is bulimia, which involves binging and purging by vomiting and laxatives.

Junk Water

Sure, fruit drinks are cheaper than pure juices when it's your turn to furnish snacks for the soccer team. The grocery store shelves are filled with a variety of colored sugar water, sold as "fruit drinks." These selections are little more than high-priced water with corn syrup and a touch of juice for flavor and color appeal.

Is this a girl's disease? No. Teen boys feel pressure to perform well in sports or need to "make weight" for sports like gymnastics or wrestling. A much smaller percentage of all eating disorders occur in males. As parents we must make ourselves aware of the warning signs for eating disorders, and research proper treatment methods. If you suspect your child has an eating disorder, partner with your pediatrician for answers and support.

Where's the Beef?

Vegetarianism is fast becoming a popular nutrition lifestyle choice. Many teens are vegetarians because their families are concerned about animal rights or religious and cultural beliefs. Others practice a meatless lifestyle by their own volition; they're vegans because it is "trendy." The benefits of a vegetarian diet are largely determined by the nutrient substitutions for meat in the diet. If teens substitute chips and candy for meat, they gain no health benefits and instead only gain empty calories of sugar and saturated fats.

Nutrients found in meat, poultry, and fish, such as calcium, iron, and vitamin B12, are scarce in a vegetarian's diet. Provide other protein sources if your family or teenager practices a meatless lifestyle. Beans, nuts, lentils, tofu, and other soy products all contain protein and meet the regulations of a vegan's diet.

- **Calcium**—Calcium is very important for healthy bones and teeth. Low calcium leads to weak bones that break easily and contributes to early tooth decay.
- **Iron**—Iron plays an important role in red blood cell formation. A lack of iron can cause some types of anemia, lowering your teen's energy level.
- **Vitamin B12**—Insufficient amounts of vitamin B12 can also lead to anemia. A low amount of vitamin B12 creates poor memory functions and weak muscles.

Losses of any of these nutrients during a teen's growth could cause a host of problems now and in their future. Teenage bodies are still strengthening bones and teeth. Teens need high amounts of energy and strong muscles to keep up with their busy lifestyles. If your teen plays sports, a vegetarian diet that is not properly monitored and supplemented might affect performance and increase the chance for injury. This is definitely not the time to start losing good muscle function!

A Sweeter Feeling

If you have an overexcited and foggy feeling following a high-sugar meal or snack, you are a sugar-sensitive person. To avoid that unfocused feeling, concentrate on eating complex carbohydrates and avoid pure carbohydrate foods. Try combo foods, those mixed with protein and low fat, such as yogurt. The fat slows the rate of stomach emptying and delays absorption of sugar into the blood. Eating raw foods rather than cooked ones also slows the absorption process.

Sunny "D"

Since teenagers still live at home and some of their lifestyle choices depend on parents, we still facilitate healthy food choices. If both parents work outside the home, teens spend more time unsupervised, and our influence on nutrition and activity choices diminishes. Since they spend so much more time inside and choose to spend their time on the computer or in front of the television, they are not exposed to natural sunlight, which stimulates the body to produce vitamin D.

All it takes is 10 minutes a day a few times a week out in the sun *without* sunscreen, plus a single glass of milk per day, to give a teen the needed amounts of vitamin D and calcium to build strong bones. Try picnic lunches on the weekends, or have your teen do some outside household chores like mowing the yard. Use multivitamins, green leafy veggies, and milk as good sources of vitamin D. Replace soft drinks with milk at mealtimes. For an added amount of vitamin D, sneak in good greens like a fresh green salad or a spinach casserole whenever you can.

Beating Burnout

Mood swings still affect a teenager's personality and range from excitement and high energy to depression. Hormones play a factor, but new responsibilities, like a part-time job and college or career planning, stress a teen's body even more. Strained relationships with family, friends, employers, or teachers can set a teen on the path to burnout. Poor eating habits only compound these otherwise-normal and expected stresses. Teens burn the candle at both ends.

Since every child is different when it comes to what will stress him out, it's important to be watchful. Is he moody or hanging around the house more than usual? Is he having trouble sleeping, or experiencing a dip—or an increase—in appetite? Has he lost interest in the activities he usually enjoys or started to struggle in school? If you see any of these changes, talk to him to find out what's upsetting him. Tell him that what matters most is his happiness.

Watch for signs of family stress, too. What we do can make things better or worse. The preparation, transportation, and juggling of daily life is your job—and sometimes it's just too much. If all the carpooling leaves you grumpy, or family dinners are a distant memory and homework is getting lost in the shuffle, it's time to rethink the schedule. Even though we want our teens to make their own schedules, many still don't know how. If it seems he's burning the candle at both ends, you need to intervene.

Keep the body in balance and moderate your child's moods with antistress foods such as apples, pears, or strawberries served with a slice of cheese. A light carbohydrate meal balanced with some protein keeps blood sugars level and can also reduce mood swings.

The best stress buster is regular exercise. Give your kids the facts about how food and exercise affect their moods. They may not seem to listen, but hopefully they'll recall some bit of the advice and act on it. Be a positive and consistent role model, and take care of yourself first by eating healthy and exercising regularly.

The Pressure Is On

Teenagers show their independence in the choices they make when they're away from you. Experimenting with "new things" and deciding for one's self is characteristic of a 15- to 18-year-old. With the pressure of peers at a teen's side, some decisions—like whether or not to try drugs—can be difficult.

Tobacco, stimulants, alcohol, and narcotics use and abuse is more common than we'd like. Teenagers sometimes use these drugs to help them "fit in" at school, lose weight, increase energy, or lift their mood. Some look for quick ways to boost energy due to fatigue from lack of sleep and busy schedules. Some turn to caffeine in the form of soda or coffee. Others turn to pills. Many girls smoke hoping to decrease their appetite so that they'll lose weight. A well-balanced diet that includes adequate protein and complex carbohydrates combats symptoms of fatigue and steadies their moods. Quick energy foods like a handful of mixed nuts, a hard-boiled egg, or tuna and cheese on wheat crackers give a boost to a tired teen.

If you think your teenager may be involved in drug use of any kind, confront your child and meet with your family doctor or counselor to deal with the situation properly.

The Four A's of Fiber

Remember the four A's of fiber: apples, artichokes, apricots, and avocados.

The Three B's of Fiber

Remember the three B's of fiber: beans, berries, and bran. One serving of bran plus one serving of beans each day will give you more than half of your total daily fiber needs. Bran and berries mixed with yogurt make for a great breakfast or snack.

Connect the Dots

Lifestyle demands, more responsibilities, and newfound freedoms affect teens' decisions about when, where, and what they eat. Part-time jobs, dating, and even a new driver's license foster independence and leave teens to feed themselves. Although this is good practice for when they eventually leave home either to go to college or to get a job and live on their own, parents can still influence teens' eating habits while they still live at home.

Teenagers' diets may not be balanced in terms of all the minerals, vitamins, and energy nutrients they need. The growth time in the teenage years bring on dramatic increases in their height and hormonal levels. Some nutrients, such as iron, are especially important with the onset of menstruation in teenage girls and the increase of lean body mass in boys. In order to convince teens that they need more quality calories filled with vitamins to match their energy requirements, they'll first have to understand the connection between how they feel and perform and what they eat.

One way to heighten their interest toward nutrition is to appeal to their intellect. All teenagers need more energy to do more things. Teenagers like to stay up later, go out with friends, play sports, and do more than schoolwork and chores. Talk to your teen about how nutrition is important when there is a change in schedule or activities. Energy needs vary depending on growth rate, body composition, and activity level. A 15-year-old girl, whose growth is nearly completed and is inactive, needs no more than 2,000 calories daily. A boy the same age, who is in a growth spurt and participates in sports, needs approximately 4,000 calories daily to retain his weight.

Fast Foods

The small intestine is in charge of food absorption. Yet, some substances, such as alcohol and caffeine, and some drugs, like aspirin, can be absorbed through the lining of the stomach—hence the tipsy or buzzlike feeling that occurs even before finishing an alcoholic drink or cup of coffee. Consuming mind-altering substances on an empty stomach increases the speed of their absorption.

Edible Energy

If a teen sleeps a lot or more than necessary and is missing out on fun activities with friends, it's time to talk about nutritional energy sources. Educate and encourage; don't demand. Just say that B vitamins give him more energy, and then ask him which veggies you should pick up at the store for him. Don't nag, and forget the guilt; just seize the moment and teach.

It's still your job to set your child up for success by providing a wide selection of healthy foods. Your teen wants to make his *own* choices, but this ensures his food choices are from quality foods. Keep a variety of quick, healthy snacks and easy-to-prepare meals on hand, so he won't feel the need to go to a drive-through. In chapters 9 through 12, we provide a plethora of recipes to choose from. The following table shows daily nutrient needs for a teenager:

Nutrient Requirements per Day

Calories	2,200 (girls); 3,000 (boys)
Protein	55 grams (girls); 66 grams (boys)
Iron	15 milligrams (girls); 11 milligrams (boys)
Calcium	1,300 milligrams
Zinc	15 milligrams
Vitamin A	2,300 IU (girls); 3,000 IU (boys)
Vitamin C	70 milligrams
Vitamin D	10 IU

We used to think that teens respond differently to the world because of hormones, or attitudes, or a simple need for independence. But now we know that their brains just actually work differently than adult brains. If we catch ourselves saying, "Use your brain!" what we don't realize is we're asking teens to use an adult brain that they have yet to develop. We expect things from them they are just not capable of giving. They're using a part of the brain that responds with reaction, not reason. But as they get older, they will depend more on the frontal cortex, which helps us read the emotions of others more accurately.

Right now we can help our kids develop their adult brains by providing them with opportunities to bring reason and logic into the picture. Over the course of a week, try to incorporate the following exercises that promote connection between mind and body. These mental calisthenics can go a long way to improve brain function by preparing it to accept learning opportunities more easily.

Mind in Motion

Movement and exercise contribute to the activation of new neurons in the brain that increase the capacity to learn. Many of our teens are too sedentary and then find themselves in a learning slump as well. If your child isn't actively involved in a sport, at least encourage her to take a brisk walk every day. In order to avoid that "do what I say and not what I do" scenario, make it a point to take 15 minutes and walk with your child. You might be surprised how it builds not only new neurons but also a better relationship between parent and child.

If your teen participates regularly in sports, make sure she takes some time every day to practice a skill related to that sport. Whether it is muscle building, endurance building, or accuracy building, encourage her to spend about 20–30 minutes engaged in this activity. Be there while she does it and act as your child's spotter, timer, or cheerleader.

Play Ball

Teens often struggle with how to study and remember information. One way to help connect movement with learning is to study using a ball that you toss back and forth and when it is again in your child's hands, he has to say the memorized fact. For example, if he is studying Greek word roots, you can say the root, toss the ball to him, and he has to provide the English meaning. Vary this exercise by using a bean bag, a soft toy, or even go outside and throw the Frisbee around. Poems, formulas, vocabulary, historical facts and dates, the Periodic Table of Elements, and even the Declaration of Independence can be recited using this exercise.

Rhythmic Breathing

Increasing blood oxygen flow circulates oxygen to the brain and increases learning. This breathing exercise can be done regularly, especially before a situation that is challenging or unpleasant or that produces some anxiety, like a test, an interview, or a ball game.

- Inhale for 8 counts.
- Hold breath for 12 counts.
- Slowly exhale for 10 counts.
- Repeat 10 times.

Tree Planting

The dendrites in our brains are like trees. They continue to branch, grow, and form new synaptic connections as we learn and experience more of the world. Lack of use causes dendrites to disappear, but even teens and adults can plant a new "tree" in its place. Encourage your child to do something completely different than she has ever done before. The goal is to stimulate the brain with new ideas, sensations, and experiences. Travel somewhere you've never gone before. Listen to music you've never heard before. Read a romance when you've only read sci-fi. Go into a shop that you usually avoid and browse. Learn a new language. Enter a contest. Learn a new craft or skill. Just make sure it is completely new. This exercise in itself promotes lifelong learning.

Copy Cat

Following directions is always an important skill no matter the age. This exercise allows your child to integrate both listening and touch to create something from following directions. Start by drawing a simple picture, and then direct your teen to draw the same picture, without showing him what you've drawn. He will follow your directions, and when finished, compare drawings. This usually brings a laugh! Most likely your directions were faulty or not specific enough. Now give him a chance to be the artist and have you draw according to his directions. Then talk about how either of you could have improved the directions you gave.

Moody Music

Music may be a big part of your teen's life. She may already spend a lot of time in her room listening to music. It's a relaxation technique she already uses. If your child has spent time studying for a big test and just wants to escape and "veg out," encourage her first to review for her test one last time with your help to music. Have her lie down still either on the floor or bed, close her eyes, and relax every muscle of her body so that she can feel herself sink into the bed. Play music that she likes but that is not distracting. Then read aloud over the music whatever it was that she was studying. Afterward, let your teen have her privacy to listen to whatever music will provide her much-needed escape.

Chapter 8

CHALLENGES TO FEEDING OUR KIDS RIGHT

A man's palate can, in time,
become accustomed to anything.
NAPOLEON BONAPARTE

Why did I volunteer to drive on this field trip? "Just say no"—easier said than done. What started out as a simple 2-hour trip to the botanical gardens was about to turn into a feeding fiasco. We were supposed to be back before lunch—now we're eating there before hustling the kids back into cars and driving an hour back home.

This changes everything. Zachery, my 9-year-old human garbage disposal, will test the limits of how much food I can pack in one lunch box—and then beg for more. Savannah, his twin sister, won't want anything. Getting her to eat away from home is like trying to get a canary to eat comfortably alongside a bunch of cats. Maybe it's because of her braces, but she hates eating in front of anyone not her family. Junie, my 2-year-old, along for the ride, is in this "French fries only" stage. Where am I going to get French fries in the middle of the botanical gardens? And then there's James. I promised his mother I would take him with us on the trip since she wasn't feeling well. I have no idea what James eats, and now I have to make a lunch for him, too.

It's supposed to be really hot, so I'll need more drinks than usual. We'll be eating outside, so I guess I need something for us all to sit on. There's obviously no refrigeration, so a large cooler is probably in order. What's easy to eat and clean up? If I can't give Junie French fries, will she just eat a handful of some cereal until we get home? Oh, wait, James is lactose intolerant, so forget the milk. But that means I have to bring juice just for him since I don't give my kids juice for lunch. And if I do give it to James, the rest will wear me out with their whining.

The morning of the trip dawned, and Carol's nerves were shot even before breakfast. Junie was up four times during the night with a fever that mysteriously disappeared with the daylight. James spent the night so his mother could rest, but he wouldn't eat their dinner and woke up at 3 A.M. complaining of hunger. It was going to be a long day. Carol surveyed the inside of her refrigerator and groaned. Where were the sandwiches she so lovingly prepared the night before? He wouldn't, she thought. But he did. Her husband snatched them for himself on his way out to work without thinking they might not be for him.

"I surrender," Carol said aloud to the kids when they reminded her they had to leave in just 5 minutes. She hurried them out the door and into the car—and stopped at Chicken King on the way to the botanical gardens.

THE BEST OF INTENTIONS

There's something to be said for convenience when it comes to feeding our kids. Even if you regularly encourage them to buy lunch at school, there will still be those days when it's up to you to feed them lunch. There are a myriad of situations that require more planning than others. Once outside the comfort of your own kitchen, things can get a little dicey. Nutrition gets sacrificed for convenience, and suddenly all the best intentions get trampled by the green-eyed monster, the ticking clock, or an empty wallet. Some situations require special handling, and learning a few food selections, preparation, and packing tips can ease both your mind and your child's hunger pains.

Even though we're concerned about our children's nutrition, many other things rival for that number one spot in our priorities. Grades, peer pressures, and safety all occupy a lot of our brain space. These issues, although important, can't be controlled as much as we'd like. What we do and say to our kids at home affects what they say and do while they're at school. Making sure hot lunch at school is good for them seems out of your control, but it doesn't have to be. We want our kids to have a nutritious lunch, but then we choose to send them to school with money to buy lunch. And if we believe that the school lunch is less nutritious, why do we do it?

Feedback

Children generally seek to please their parents. Pass out the praise for making wise food choices and experimenting with new taste sensations.

Making Wise Choices

Convenience is the unlabeled ingredient in most of the foods we choose for ourselves and our kids. We can tell it's convenient by its preparation (less prep time in the morning and doesn't need to be heated), its packaging (juice box or thermos; a boxed meal or homemade sandwich), and if it's "tasty" (kids won't complain and they'll actually eat it).

Convenience isn't just for kid food; as adults we eat that way, too. But choosing only what's convenient comes with a price if we don't choose wisely. What impact do your own eating habits have on your kids? If you demand they have protein for breakfast, yet you skip breakfast all together, what does that tell them? Convenience and nutrition can go hand in hand. If we spend more time now, we can spend less time later. Prepare healthy choices in easy-to-grab portions ahead of time, and you won't get caught empty handed running out the door. A thermos full of a yogurt smoothie, a baggie of granola or trail mix, and even a small container or zipped bag of bite-size fruits or veggies combine convenience with good nutrition.

Kitchen Helpers

Give your child opportunities to learn about food by helping out in the kitchen. Kids are more likely to eat what they helped cook.

What's in Your Bag?

Kids sometimes judge what they have for lunch. Sometimes the reason nutrition goes out the window is because our kids see something "better" in their friend's lunch box. Sometimes kids trade lunches because they don't have the popular snack that everyone else seems to have. And sometimes they're embarrassed by their own lunch. Vicki's son won't bring his lunch to school in anything but a plastic bag. It wouldn't be "cool" to bring an insulated bag or lunch box. What happens when he finds carrot sticks, a tuna sandwich on wheat bread, a plum, and a thermos full of milk in his lunch box, but his best friend has a burrito, fruit roll-ups, chips, and a blue raspberry juice pouch in theirs? Trading.

Trading happens whether you send him with a healthy lunch or not. Sometimes someone else's food looks better. "I'll give you my gummy worms for your sour blasters," "If you give me half of your personal pizza, I'll give you my chocolate chip cookies," or even "How much do you want for your soda?" This is a form of peer pressure, to be sure. No one wants to be made fun of for what they eat, but it happens all the time. Our kids need to learn what's right and eat what's right regardless of what their friends eat. And for parents, we need to feed our kids the right things regardless of what other parents feed their kids. The challenges to getting our kids to eat right never seem to end!

Add Your Own Oats

If you are eating oat bran for your heart or bowels, rather than looking for small amounts added to cereals such as granola, buy a package of oat bran and sprinkle it on your choice of cereal.

How Much Does It Cost?

Family finances do play a role in what we feed our kids. Buying lunch at school is more expensive, so some parents opt to pack their child's own lunch. There are families for whom even this is a hardship. That's why the National School Lunch Program exists—to ensure that children from impoverished homes get an adequate breakfast and lunch at school each day. Regardless of your income level, you can send your kids to school with a nutritious lunch that's affordable, but you may have to first change your buying habits. Here are some money-saving tips if you're looking for a way to trim your budget without skimping on nutrition.

- **Avoid snacks and juices marketed just for kids.** They are often more expensive and tend to have higher amounts of sugar. You can buy concentrated juices and full-size snacks and then package them yourself into kid-size containers or baggies. Buy canned fruit packed in water if fresh fruit is too expensive or not in season, and spoon into small containers instead of buying fruit roll-ups or fruit snacks.

- **Buy fruits and veggies uncut and prepare them yourself.** Fresh fruit or cut-up veggies make great snacks and cost less than prepackaged foods. Buy them uncut and then cut them into bite-size pieces at home yourself.
- **Water down your juice.** Most juices still have too much sugar in them and cost more than most of us want to spend. Dilute your children's juice with ⅓ to ½ cup of water. Flavor will not be compromised, and neither will your child's weight and dental health.
- **Don't buy your favorite cookie.** If you choose to buy cookies instead of making them yourself, buy a cookie that you like, not love. Kids will still eat them but won't go through them as quickly. Try to buy cookies on sale.
- **Buy store brands.** If you choose to buy chips, pretzels, and cookies for your kids' lunches, buy the store brand instead of the name brand. Kids won't really notice, and if they do, they'll eat the store brand chips rather than no chips at all. Store brands often go on sale, and in-store coupons make them that much more attractive to savvy shoppers.

IT'S TIME FOR A CHANGE

Believe it or not, many sack lunches made at home fail to provide a balanced, nutritious meal. Moms pack more foods containing partially hydrogenated oils, sugars, and salt and less foods containing vegetables (sources of fiber), vitamins, and antioxidants than they did 20 years ago. The following changes will make a tremendous impact on your child's eating habits:

- Most kids bring sandwiches for lunch at school—two-thirds of those are made on white bread. *Nutritious change*: substitute light wheat or whole wheat bread.
- Meat sandwiches, like bologna, are the most common, followed by peanut butter and jelly. *Nutritious change*: buy meat from the deli; use organic peanut butter and preserves instead of jelly.

- Girls get vegetables in their lunches almost twice as often as boys. At the same age (8–11 years old), girls start bringing more salads and boys start bringing more cake. *Nutritious change*: buy salad fixings that your kids can choose from themselves and pack in their own lunch.
- Sweet snacks are included in most homemade lunches at least once a week, with cookies surpassing all other sweets. *Nutritious change*: Combat childhood obesity by limiting the sweets. If you include cookies, try making them yourself to reduce or even eliminate the sugar and salt intake.

Even when we take complete responsibility for what our kids eat for lunch, it isn't perfect. There will be weeks when your schedule just doesn't allow for perfect planning. There will be paychecks too small to promote perfect food selection. And there will be family health issues that thwart your attempts to get anything of substance into your child (whether you're sick or they are). The goal is to more often than not feed your children nutrient-rich foods. Some days will be better than others. Look at how your child ate over the course of a week, and see if you are satisfied that it balanced itself out. Everything in moderation!

Buzz Foods

Some foods, such as those that contain caffeine, give the brain a buzz—a welcome lift when the brain needs to be turned on. Other times caffeinated foods can be an obstacle to sleep and relaxation.

EATING INSIDE, OUTSIDE, UPSIDE DOWN

We don't always have control over what our children eat since we can't be with them every hour of every day. Whether our child attends a public, private, or home school, the logistics may demand flexibility on our part. Special occasions, holidays, or outings also test our creativity when it comes to feeding our kids. And sometimes someone else will choose what our children eat when they go to someone else's house. These are all challenges to making sure kids eat right when they're away from us. Be aware of the advantages and pitfalls of each situation. That way if where they eat doesn't provide the healthiest meals, you can balance out your kid's nutrition during a time when you are together.

Eating at a Public School

Each type of schooling creates its own set of unique feeding challenges. If your child attends public school, you might disagree with menu choices and question their nutrition value. But there are advantages to eating in a public school. If you need financial assistance, your child can eat breakfast and lunch either at a reduced price or for free. If you leave for work very early in the morning, your child can take advantage of a school breakfast program before school starts. Because public schools fall under the jurisdiction of state and federal control, they are required to follow federal dietary guidelines and make breakfast and lunch affordable to all children who need it.

Public schools also try to provide snacks for those children who participate in some sort of after-school program (e.g., the YMCA) until they're picked up later in the evening. More recently, public schools also have started to provide nutritious snacks during fall and spring testing times to help kids concentrate better on tests. The PTA often takes on this responsibility.

Eating at a Private School

Private schools, including those affiliated with churches, are a different story. Some have full kitchens and provide hot lunches, but many don't. More often there's a bank of microwaves lining a counter for students to use to warm up something they brought from home. Often some of these schools will sponsor a "pizza day" when pizza is brought in from a local restaurant and parents volunteer to serve it to the kids. Some private schools do participate in the national lunch program and are subsidized and receive commodities, but most don't. Since some parents have to work extra hard to afford to send their kids to a private school, they may still find it difficult to afford lunch. Unfortunately, they don't receive any sort of benefits and still must provide their own breakfast and lunch.

If parent involvement is high, there are ways to provide more meals for kids. Since there is no budget for food service workers, parents may choose to fill in that gap to prepare meals, supervise children, and double as a custodial staff to clean up afterward. It's a rare school, however, that has parents willing to take the time to do these tasks.

Eating at Home

One advantage of homeschooling would seem to include being able to make sure your child eats three nutritious meals per day. This isn't always the case. Homeschool moms find themselves just as busy as their traditional school counterparts. In an attempt to provide a well-rounded educational experience for their kids, they attend enrichment classes, go on frequent field trips, and volunteer as a family in their communities. That equals an awful lot of lunches away from home, and eating in the car is a common detour of their daily commutes.

No matter where your kids go to school, you can take control of their health. Parents all over the country gather together to promote student wellness by joining the school committees that make goals for nutrition education and physical activity a priority. Parents with children who attend private schools can also spearhead the responsibility to combat childhood obesity (if it's something they're faced with as a family) and a sedentary lifestyle by insisting on more nutritious food when it is served and more physical activity as a regular part of the school day through their governing boards. Homeschool parents can educate their own families through personal study and by planning and shopping for meals with their children. All families can do that, but homeschool parents can easily integrate these activities into their curricula. Even when our kids eat breakfast and lunch somewhere else, we can help them to make wise choices by first modeling those choices for them and providing healthy choices when they're at home.

Hot Foods for Colds

Hot, spicy foods such as chili peppers, hot mustard, radishes, pepper, onions, and garlic contain substances called *mucolytics* that liquefy thick mucus that accumulates in the sinuses and breathing passages (similar to over-the-counter expectorant cough syrups).

School Parties and Holidays

"Mom, I need to bring in some kind of food to celebrate Cinco de Mayo in Spanish tomorrow!" Food and school tend to go together. Teachers love to incorporate food into their lessons whenever possible and when they're brave enough. When a teacher decides to make a lesson more relevant by including food, this isn't a "fun" day—no matter what kids think. It is more work before, during, and after than any other day. Parents don't think of it as "fun," either. Their jobs include the selecting, purchasing, preparing, and transporting of the "special" food to school.

As much work as this is for parents and teachers, and as much fun as it is for kids to eat, these "special" foods can be nutritious too. There are always those who send in a bag of chips they picked up at the last minute on the way to school or those who prefer just to provide the paper products, but for those who actually commit to making the green chile enchiladas, Irish stew, red beans and rice, or even the crispy rice treats for Halloween, consider these suggestions:

- **Prepare something that does not require reheating**. A classroom is no place for a dozen crock pots, and the microwave is usually across the school in the teacher's lounge.
- **Choose a recipe that has simple and identifiable ingredients**. Anything too complicated promises to include something someone has either an allergy to or an intolerance of. Label your meal with a short list of ingredients to avoid "I wonder what's in that."
- **Low-sugar the sweets**. If you are charged with bringing some kind of dessert, choose a recipe with little to no sugar or a natural substitute like applesauce. Kids (and their teachers) don't need a sugar high. They have enough energy on their own.
- **Plan on sticking around if you have time**. The older kids get, the fewer the parents that help out in the schools. Even if you weren't able to prepare food for the fiesta, volunteer to chaperone the event and help clean up afterward. Monitor what and how much the kids eat. Encourage them to try something they've never had before. Caution those who take more than their share. Then take charge of cleaning up so the teacher can get back to what she does best—teach.

Holidays and special occasions celebrated at school, when coupled with food, make a lasting impression on kids. They provide those all-important brain connections that transfer an experience into long-term memory.

Out and About

It seems that we all spend more time eating somewhere other than our own dining room tables. How many drive-throughs do you frequent on a weekly basis? But fast food isn't the only family dinnertime thief. Our children eat out during school, church, sports, and club outings;

they eat over at their friends' houses. Although these activities add spice to our kids' lives, we don't want them to get heartburn! An overindulgence of eating out steals precious moments away from family togetherness, valuable training time, and homework time.

Try It, You Might Like It!

Have children and parents take turns choosing a new food to introduce to the family.

WHAT DO YOU LEARN AT THE DINNER TABLE?

Mealtime conversation marries nutritional and learning needs. Although "What did you do in school today?" is most commonly served, there are topical side dishes you can try. Sometimes families find themselves saving the frustrations or disappointments of the day for the dinner table. But that's like only serving Brussels sprouts for the main course (apologies to those who love Brussels sprouts). If dinnertime becomes a time of strife or anxiety, we'll avoid it and will make no real connections. If it's enjoyable and relaxing, both the body and the mind will be fed. Consider these mealtime guidelines:

- **When everyone is home, require the family to sit at the table together.** Sometimes even when we're all home, everyone finds a different spot to eat: Dad in front of the television, kids in the family room, and Mom in the kitchen alone. Gather around the table together, not just to avoid messes all over the house but to focus on one another.
- **Don't discipline at the dinner table.** Even if something went wrong at school or at home, deal with the infraction after dinner. Try not to associate eating together with negative experiences. Don't dish out punishments during mealtimes. If you have to address the issue, do so briefly and set a time after dinner to deal with it completely.
- **How was your day?** As adults, ask one another how your day was and whether anything new or interesting happened. Kids learn about the pitfalls and pleasures of your day and will become more willing to share about their own days. This also gives them an opportunity

to discover how you handled things that went wrong. These are teachable moments. How about asking the kids directly about their day? Take turns to answer "What was the *best* part of your day? And what was the *worst* part of your day?" You'll learn a lot.

■ **Encourage inclusive conversation**. Sometimes certain family members tend to monopolize dinnertime conversation. It's fine to briefly talk about things that are only of interest to one or two members, but when possible, try to choose topics that engage all those sitting around the table. Not only is this a great way to make sure no one feels left out, but it nurtures mealtime etiquette that children will need in future social settings.

Studies show that kids who eat more family meals perform better in school. They spend more time on homework, get better grades, and spend more of their free time reading for pleasure. But there are other benefits, too. Eating together at home saves time. Eating out may save effort, but it takes more time than eating at home. Kids have homework to do on a regular basis, and as parents, we need to protect that time. They're already so busy with extracurricular activities, sports, church, and friends. School must come first if they are going to succeed. We can set them up for success by setting the dinner table as a family as often as possible.

more mouths to feed

Once in a while you'll have more mouths to feed than usual. It changes the way you do things. It changes what you choose to serve. It changes your focus on nutrition. It can derail your wellness efforts if you let it. If you discover other people's children sitting around your table, you might alter your normal selections in favor of more kid-friendly food. And when the lazy, hazy days of summer come and everyone is home for every meal more regularly, you may get lazy yourself and stock up on fun, frozen foods that kids can make for themselves. The challenge is not to walk away from the good habits you've already established when you hit a bump in the road. Healthy eating and brain function don't take a holiday.

A Newcomer's Needs

A major life change, like having a baby or bringing in an elderly parent to live with you, challenges you to prepare foods to meet their preferences and needs. There are some dietary needs specific to these age groups, but try not to sacrifice the rest of your family's nutritional needs in favor of the newcomer's. You may find that your time is more limited caring for a newborn or elderly parent. Both have dietary restrictions. Both may require assistance in the actual feeding process. Both have brains that depend on good nutrition. The upside to preparing meals for both these groups is that their nutritional needs can positively influence the rest of the family's eating habits. As babies grow and are able to eat table food, it's best that they eat foods with no preservatives, simple sugars, or excess salt. That's good for everyone! Your elderly father may be diabetic, have cardiovascular illnesses or Alzheimer's, and follow a specially recommended diet that actually contributes to the wellness of the entire family. The heightened nutrition awareness that comes with caring for these extra mouths forces families to learn what is and isn't good for them to eat. When children understand the real-life impact certain foods have on their overall health and learning, they are less likely to fight you on your food choices.

Can Jimmy Eat Over?

Do you cringe when your child asks if a friend can eat lunch or dinner at your house? Do you panic when one of their friends spends the night and you're faced with feeding a complete stranger breakfast in the morning? Do you run out to the store to buy frozen chicken fingers, curly fries, soda, and cookie dough? Or do you punch the speed dial on your phone and order from Pizza House? Too many of us fear rejection by these "little" people and make changes to our existing mealtime routines just to please them. Consistency is the key. Let your kids' friends see what it's like to live and eat in your house. Even if they don't like what you serve that night, they will see a family that enjoys eating together and values good nutrition. For all you know, what they eat at your house may be the only nutritious meal they'll eat all week. You can contribute to another child's well-being and development by not deviating from the balanced approach you use to feed your own kids.

Summertime and the Breakfast Is Skipped

When kids are in school, at least one of their meals may be taken care of. If they eat breakfast at school, too, then you only have to plan for dinner. But during the summer those numbers may increase to two or three meals per day. We have to be just as diligent to make sure they eat right. Many kids don't eat breakfast at all during the school year, so summer is a chance to instill this all-important habit. For some reason, breakfast tends to get sidestepped in the summer. Kids tend to sleep in longer, and teens may miss the breakfast hour(s) all together. When kids do wake up, they may plop themselves immediately in front of the television (a luxury they probably didn't have during the school year) and cruise right through breakfast. "Summertime and the livin' is lazy" is more like it. For those of us who work full-time out of the home, the routine is the same. But for those of us who work at home, the opportunity to make sure our kids eat three good meals per day is not always a welcome one.

Breakfast is still the most important meal of the day, even in the summer. Pediatricians agree that children who eat breakfast regularly think faster and clearer, solve problems more easily, and are less likely to be irritable. That makes for a more pleasant child to live with for 24 hours a day during the summer. Establishing good eating habits begins with breakfast. Welcome this summer as an opportunity to retrain your entire family in the art of breakfast. There's more to life than cereal or frozen waffles. There are menu suggestions and recipes for breakfast at the end of this book to get you started. If you want to take control of one meal, this is the one to put your energy into. Keep these tips in mind to entice your child to eat breakfast every day:

- **Plan a weekly breakfast menu together**. Even if they choose to have the same thing every day, encourage them to choose something else for the following week. The idea is to experiment with different foods to see if kids like them and to gauge how much time and effort they take to prepare in anticipation for the following school year.
- **Turn off the television**. Expect your children to eat breakfast with you at the table. Use this time to go over the plans for the day.
- **Eat breakfast yourself**. Often we find ourselves downing only a cup of coffee or skipping breakfast altogether while we expect our kids to eat a full meal at breakfast. For your own health and to be a good role model, sit down with your children and eat!
- **Make it easy**. Keep breakfast foods visible and accessible for kids. Try to put dried fruits, granola bars, mixed nuts, and cereals on a bottom shelf. Have at least three easy-to-serve items that

are good for them available for those who are old enough to make their own breakfast. See the section on breakfast in chapter 9.

Summer eating goes hand in hand with summer learning. We become lazy learners during the summer and lazy eaters. It takes some effort on our parts to create better eating and learning habits in our kids over the summer, but not as much effort as it will be to break them of bad habits during the school year.

Unfortunately, many kids forget some of what they've learned, and by the end of the summer they lose more than two and a half months of grade-level equivalency. Teachers may spend up to 6 weeks at the beginning of every school year trying to review what the kids learned at the end of the last school year. Waste of time. In order to combat learning loss, we can beef up both our children's nutrient intake and their educational intake. Skills are just a set of habits, and new habits can be formed over a 30-day period. Summer is a great time to instill new and improved eating and learning habits in our kids.

Rank the Breads

As with grains, ranking breads is difficult. Here we rate breads according to nutrients such as protein, fiber, calcium, iron, zinc, folic acid, niacin, riboflavin, and vitamins B6 and E from best to worst:

1. **Multi–whole grain**
2. **Whole wheat**
3. **Pita, whole wheat**
4. **Pumpernickel**
5. **Rye, American**
6. **White**

WISE CHOICES FOR WELLNESS

The challenges to feed our kids right seem neverending. We battle outside influences. We play tug-of-war with their tastes and preferences. We fight our own attraction toward the convenience monster. And sometimes we just plain give up too easily. But the battle for our kids' wellness is worth fighting. What we put into them today comes out in life later on. The habits we instill now will carry them through their own adulthoods and into the lives of our grandchildren. Each challenge is an opportunity to make the right choices—again.

PART III

recipes for success

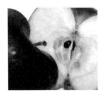 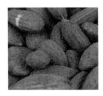 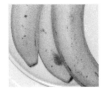

Chapter 9

Breakfast: eye openers

Breakfast, we've all heard, is the most important meal of the day, but why? What's the big deal about breakfast? Breakfast does magic for our bodies because it gives our bodies fuel and energy to start the day. It also is the first meal we eat after an 8- to 12-hour fast since we last ate dinner or an evening snack. Every morning you have an opportunity to start your body right by choosing to eat a balanced breakfast before racing out the door.

Our bodies are like cars. What do we put in a car to make it run? What would happen if we put juice or milk into the car? The car needs its special kind of fuel. Our bodies are the same. We must put the right kind of fuel into our bodies if we want them to work correctly. If your

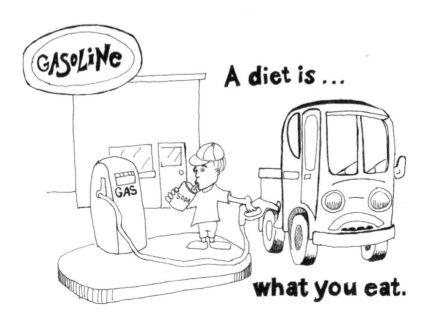

body doesn't have fuel (food), it will not be able to move and do the activities you need to do. Just as a car with a gas tank low on fuel won't run smoothly and will have trouble starting, when your body does not have food to start the day, it feels slow and tired from the get-go.

Almost any healthy food can be a breakfast food. The best breakfast is a combination of foods that supply protein, fat, and carbohydrates to sustain energy and concentration for several hours. Providing a choice of foods from at least three food groups gives children and teenagers the nutrients and energy they need to feel good and do well in school. For children and adults, balanced breakfast choices help provide the healthy edge needed for optimum health and academic performance.

Here are a few quick meals that include at least three food groups. More recipes and breakfast meal suggestions follow. Eat and be happy!

Quick No-Cook Balanced Meal Suggestions
- Cheese rolled over a breadstick and a glass of fruit juice
- Toast with frozen fruit and a glass of milk
- Toaster waffles with a banana and glass of milk
- Bananas rolled in vanilla yogurt and granola
- Cereal with milk and fruit
- Whole wheat toast spread with peanut butter and 100 percent fruit spread
- Fruit smoothie made with milk or yogurt and fresh fruit

Breakfast cone

Ingredients

1 plain ice cream cone

¼ cup fat-free yogurt

¼ cup sliced fruit of choice

2 tablespoons crunchy cereal

Step 1: Add fruit to yogurt; mix.

Step 2: Pour yogurt mixture into ice cream cone; top with cereal.

NUTRITION

Amount per serving

Servings: 1

Calories: 124

Fat calories: 0

Percent values: 0% fat, 55% protein, 45% carb

applesauce oatmeal

Ingredients

1 package instant oatmeal, any flavor

$\frac{1}{2}$ cup applesauce

Step 1: Prepare oatmeal as directed; add applesauce; stir.

NUTRITION
Amount per serving
Servings: 1
Calories: 164
Fat calories: 41
Percent values: 25% fat, 41% protein, 34% carb

mexican omelet

Ingredients

2 large egg whites

$\frac{1}{2}$ cup frozen vegetables

$\frac{1}{4}$ cup grated low-fat cheese

2 tablespoons salsa

Nonstick cooking spray

Step 1: Heat vegetables in microwave until warm.

Step 2: Cook egg whites in skillet with cooking spray.

Step 3: Top eggs with salsa; place vegetables on top; sprinkle with cheese.

Fold in half; serve warm.

NUTRITION

Amount per serving

Servings: 1

Calories: 137

Fat calories: 45

Percent values: 33% fat, 44% protein, 23% carb

PB&B Breakfast Sandwich

Ingredients

2 slices whole wheat bread

1 tablespoon reduced-fat peanut butter

$\frac{1}{2}$ banana, thinly sliced

Step 1: Toast bread; smooth on peanut butter.

Step 2: Top with thinly sliced bananas.

NUTRITION
Amount per serving
Servings: 1
Calories: 107
Fat calories: 58
Percent values: 29% fat, 15% protein, 56% carb

STRING CHEESE BREAKFAST

PREP TIME: 5 MINUTES

Ingredients

1 stick string cheese, any flavor

6 slices (1 serving) low-fat deli meat

1 slice whole wheat bread

Step 1: Roll meat slices around cheese stick; wrap with the bread.

NUTRITION

Amount per serving

Servings: 1

Calories: 174

Fat calories: 49

Percent values: 28% fat, 39% protein, 33% carb

cantaloupe fruit bowl

Ingredients

$\frac{1}{2}$ small cantaloupe

$\frac{1}{2}$ cup fat-free yogurt

$\frac{1}{2}$ cup pineapple chunks in juice

Step 1: Halve cantaloupe and scoop out seeds.

Step 2: Spoon yogurt into cantaloupe half; top with pineapple chunks, drained.

NUTRITION
Amount per serving
Servings: 2
Calories: 236
Fat calories: 0
Percent values: 0% fat, 27% protein, 73% carb

Breakfast Bagel

Ingredients

1 whole wheat bagel

2 tablespoons fat-free cream cheese

2 tablespoons 100 percent fruit preserves

Step 1: Toast bagel; top with cream cheese and fruit.

NUTRITION

Amount per serving

Servings: 1

Calories: 153

Fat calories: 9

Percent values: 0.5% fat, 16% protein, 83% carb

Breakfast Pita

PREP TIME: 20 MINUTES

Ingredients

2 egg whites

1 tablespoon salsa

$1/4$ cup frozen vegetables

$1/4$ cup lean ham or turkey cubes

$1/4$ cup grated low-fat cheese

1 whole wheat pita, cut in halves

Step 1: Cook egg whites in microwave for 1 to 2 minutes; set aside.

Step 2: Heat frozen vegetables, meat chunks, cheese, and salsa together in a medium bowl in the microwave for 2 minutes.

Step 3: Add mixture to eggs; place in pita halves.

NUTRITION

Amount per serving

Servings: 2

Calories: 188

Fat calories: 39

Percent values: 22% fat, 43% protein, 35% carb

BLueBerry Bran muffins

Ingredients

$1\frac{1}{3}$ cups bran cereal

$\frac{3}{4}$ cup fat-free milk

$\frac{1}{4}$ cup egg substitute

2 teaspoons vanilla

1 cup flour

$\frac{1}{3}$ cup firmly packed light brown sugar

1 tablespoon baking powder

1 tablespoon baking soda

$\frac{3}{4}$ teaspoon cinnamon

$\frac{3}{4}$ cup fresh or frozen blueberries

Step 1: In a medium-size mixing bowl, combine bran cereal, milk, egg substitute, and vanilla.

Step 2: In a large bowl, combine flour, brown sugar, baking powder, baking soda, and cinnamon.

Step 3: Add cereal mixture to flour mixture and mix well.

Step 4: Add blueberries; spoon into paper-lined muffin tins, and bake for 30 minutes at 325 degrees until muffins are slightly browned.

NUTRITION
Amount per serving
Servings: 8
Calories: 161
Fat calories: 9
Percent values: 0.6% fat, 34% protein, 75% carb

breakfast kabobs

Ingredients

2 cups plain yogurt

4 tablespoons honey

1 (12 oz.) package mini frozen turkey sausage links

1 medium cantaloupe, peeled, seeded, and cut into 1-inch cubes

1 small bunch of seedless grapes

1 pint of strawberries, cut into halves

2 medium red apples, cored, peeled, and cut into 1-inch cubes

Step 1: Combine yogurt and honey in small bowl; refrigerate until ready to serve.

Step 2: Cook sausage over medium heat in skillet until browned. Drain on paper towels; cut each link in half.

Step 3: Alternately place sausage and fruit on wooden skewers.

Step 4: Serve with yogurt sauce for dipping.

NUTRITION
Amount per serving
Servings: 7
Calories: 257
Fat calories: 82
Percent values: 32% fat, 14% protein, 54% carb

Breakfast Pizza

Ingredients

10-ounce can refrigerated pizza crust

8 eggs

$\frac{1}{4}$ cup half and half

$\frac{1}{8}$ teaspoon salt

$\frac{1}{8}$ teaspoon pepper

2 tablespoons butter

8-ounce container cream cheese

8 slices cooked bacon

Step 1: Heat oven to 425 degrees. Grease a 12-inch pizza pan. Unroll dough; place on greased pan. Press out dough from center with hands. Bake for 7 minutes until crust browns.

Step 2: In a medium bowl, mix eggs, half and half, salt, and pepper; beat well. In large skillet, melt butter. Add egg mix; cook and stir until cooked through but moist. Remove from heat.

Step 3: Spoon cooked egg mix over baked crust. Drop cream cheese over the eggs. Place bacon on top of pizza.

Step 4: Bake for additional 10 minutes until crust is a golden brown.

NUTRITION

Amount per serving

Servings: 6

Calories: 305

Fat calories: 107

Percent values: 35% fat, 31% protein, 34% carb

oatmeal pancakes

Ingredients

2 eggs

2 tablespoons oil

1 cup flour

1 cup rolled oats

1½ teaspoons baking powder

½ teaspoon salt

¾ cup orange juice

½ cup fruit or nuts

2 tablespoons butter

Step 1: In a small bowl, mix eggs and oil. In a medium bowl, combine all dry ingredients.

Step 2: Stir egg mixture into dry mix, and then stir in orange juice to make a thick batter.

Add nuts or fruit.

Step 3: Heat butter in large frying pan, and then pour batter into the pan by ¼ cupfuls. Turn once when bubbling. Cook until done.

NUTRITION
Amount per serving
Servings: 9
Calories: 149
Fat calories: 46
Percent values: 31% fat, 15% protein, 54% carb

STRAWBERRY AND BANANA FRENCH TOAST

Ingredients

1 loaf (12 inches) French bread

4 ounces cream cheese, softened

$^1/_4$ cup chopped strawberries

$^1/_4$ cup chopped bananas

2 tablespoons strawberry jam

6 eggs, lightly beaten

$^3/_4$ cup milk

3 tablespoons butter

Step 1: Cut bread into eight 1$^1/_2$-inch-thick slices. Make a pocket in each slice at the top.

Step 2: Combine cream cheese, strawberries, bananas, and jam in small bowl for filling.

Step 3: Place a heaping tablespoon of filling into each pocket. Press sides of bread together after filling.

Step 4: Beat eggs and milk in wide shallow bowl. Coat each side of bread in egg mixture.

Step 5: Heat 2 tablespoons butter in large skillet over medium heat. Add bread slices; cook until light brown. Turn and cook other side. Remove and keep warm. Repeat with remaining butter and bread slices.

NUTRITION

Amount per serving

Servings: 8

Calories: 262

Fat calories: 75

Percent values: 29% fat, 14% protein, 57% carb

sunrise pizza

Ingredients

2 small bananas, peeled

4 frozen wheat waffles

$1/2$ cup low-fat whipped cream cheese

1 can (11 ounces) mandarin oranges, drained

2 teaspoons honey

Dash of ground cinnamon

Fresh berries to garnish

Step 1: Thinly slice bananas on diagonal.

Step 2: Prepare waffles according to package directions.

Step 3: Spread waffle with cream cheese. Arrange banana slices on top, overlapping.

Step 4: Arrange orange segments in the center of each pizza. Drizzle with honey. Sprinkle with cinnamon. Top with berries.

NUTRITION
Amount per serving
Servings: 4
Calories: 223
Fat calories: 36
Percent values: 16% fat, 7% protein, 77% carb

Breakfast Blossoms

Ingredients

1 (12-ounce) can buttermilk biscuits

$^3/_4$ cup strawberry preserves

$^1/_4$ teaspoon ground cinnamon

$^1/_4$ teaspoon ground nutmeg

Step 1: Grease ten 3-inch muffin cups. Separate dough into 10 biscuits. Separate each biscuit into three even sections. Place the three sections in a muffin cup, overlapping slightly. Press dough edges firmly together.

Step 2: Combine preserves, cinnamon, and nutmeg; place a tablespoon full in center of each cup.

Step 3: Bake at 375 degrees for 10 to 12 minutes or until lightly browned. Cool slightly before removing from pan. Serve warm.

NUTRITION

Amount per serving

Servings: 10

Calories: 116

Fat calories: 43

Percent values: 35% fat, 20% protein, 45% carb

cereal trail mix

Ingredients

$^1/_4$ cup butter

2 tablespoons sugar

1 teaspoon ground cinnamon

1 cup bite-size oat cereal squares

1 cup bite-size wheat cereal squares

1 cup bite-size rice cereal squares

$^1/_4$ cup toasted slivered almonds

$^3/_4$ cup raisins

Step 1: Melt butter at high for $1^1/_2$ minutes in large microwavable bowl. Add sugar and cinnamon; mix well. Add cereal and nuts; stir to coat completely.

Step 2: Microwave at high for 2 minutes. Stir well. Microwave 2 minutes more; stir well. Add raisins. Microwave an additional 2 to 3 minutes, stirring well after 2 minutes.

Step 3: Spread on paper towels; mix will become crisp as it cools. Store in an airtight container.

NUTRITION
Amount per serving
Servings: 4
Calories: 345
Fat calories: 144
Percent values: 42% fat, 11% protein, 47% carb

on-the-run smoothie

Ingredients

3 cups milk

2 cups nonfat yogurt

1 banana

1 cup frozen blueberries

$^1/_2$ cup frozen strawberries

2 tablespoons flax oil

2 tablespoons peanut butter

1 tablespoon cinnamon

Step 1: Combine all the ingredients and blend until smooth. Serve immediately.

NUTRITION
Amount per serving
Servings: 4
Calories: 223
Fat calories: 60
Percent values: 27% fat, 22% protein, 51% carb

peanut butter and banana smoothie

PREP TIME: 10 MINUTES

Ingredients

$1/_2$ banana

$1/_2$ cup low-fat vanilla yogurt

1 tablespoon peanut butter

$1/_2$ cup ice cubes

Step 1: Peel and slice banana and place in blender.

Step 2: Add yogurt, peanut butter, and ice cubes; blend until smooth and creamy. Serve.

NUTRITION
Amount per serving
Servings: 1
Calories: 188
Fat calories: 72
Percent values: 38% fat, 21% protein, 51% carb

strawberry waffle stacks

Ingredients

3 fat-free frozen waffles

4 tablespoons low-fat strawberry-flavored cream cheese

1 1/2 cup strawberry preserves

1 cup sliced strawberries

1 medium banana, sliced lengthwise

Step 1: Toast waffles according to package directions. Cut each waffle into three strips.

Step 2: Spread with strawberry-flavored cream cheese first, and then spread with the strawberry preserves.

Step 3: Top each stick with a lengthwise-cut banana slice and strawberry halves.

NUTRITION

Amount per serving

Servings: 2

Calories: 443

Fat calories: 72

Percent values: 16% fat, 38% protein, 46% carb

Chapter 10

LUNCH:
THE LUNCH BUNCH

WHAT'S THE LOWDOWN on lunch? It's a given that whether your kids eat lunch at home, school, or a friend's house, you want it to be healthy. What's not so obvious is why lunch is so important. It's *only* one meal out of the day, after all. Lunchtime is "refuel time." By the time the clock strikes 12, you begin to hear the rumbling of tummies. For those who didn't eat breakfast, lunch becomes brunch, a meal later than breakfast but earlier than lunch. Or they stick with the hunger pangs a little longer until they are not only hungry but tired, too.

Lunch gets us through our wakeful day. The food from breakfast is gone and used up in your body by the time your lunch break rolls around. Just as a car runs out of gas after a while, our body does, too. For a car, you pull up to the gas station, refill, and then you're back on the road. For us, we stop and eat lunch, and then we're back in business. Hopefully, you put enough fuel back in your tank to make it to your destination. Our destination is dinner. Here are some yummy lunch recipes that will keep your tank full. *Mangia!*

Ham Melts

Ingredients

1 tin tray ready-made dinner rolls

8 ounces Swiss cheese, sliced

8 ounces honey ham, sliced

$\frac{1}{2}$ cup brown sugar

2 tablespoons spicy mustard

2 tablespoons Heinz 57 sauce

2 tablespoons butter, melted

Step 1: Cut open the dinner rolls in half. Leave the bottom half in the tin tray.

Step 2: Place a single layer of Swiss cheese on top of the cut rolls in the tin tray.

Next, place a single layer of honey ham.

Step 3: Top with the top half of the dinner rolls.

Step 4: In a small bowl, mix together brown sugar, mustard, Heinz 57, and melted butter. Pour over the dinner rolls.

Step 5: Cover with aluminum foil. Bake at 350 degrees for 15 minutes. Uncover and cook an additional 10 minutes.

NUTRITION
Amount per serving
Servings: 6
Calories: 316
Fat calories: 117
Percent values: 38% fat, 22% protein, 40% carb

TIC TAC TOE

Ingredients

$\frac{1}{2}$ whole wheat pita stuffed with low-fat chicken salad

$\frac{1}{4}$ cup raisins

$\frac{1}{4}$ cup crunchy cereal

1 cup broccoli and cauliflower florets

$\frac{1}{4}$ cup ranch dressing for dip

3×5 index card

Step 1: On the index card, draw a Tic Tac Toe board. Let your child enjoy a game of Tic Tac Toe with friends while eating lunch, using the raisins and cereal pieces as the X's and O's.

NUTRITION
Amount per serving
Servings: 1
Calories: 321
Fat calories: 81
Percent values: 25% fat, 1% protein, 74% carb

Buffalo-Style Wraps

Ingredients

⅔ cup cayenne pepper sauce

1 tablespoon vegetable oil

4 boneless skinless chicken breast halves

¼ cup blue cheese salad dressing

1 cup shredded lettuce

1 cup shredded Monterey Jack cheese

4 (10-inch) flour tortillas, heated

Step 1: Combine ⅓ cup sauce and 1 tablespoon oil in a resealable plastic food storage bag. Add chicken. Seal bag; toss to coat evenly. Marinate in refrigerator 30 minutes or overnight.

Step 2: Broil or grill chicken 10 to 15 minutes or until no longer pink in center. Slice chicken into long thin strips. In bowl, toss chicken with remaining ⅓ cup sauce and dressing.

Step 3: Arrange chicken, lettuce, and cheese down center of tortillas, dividing evenly. Fold bottom third of each tortilla over filling; fold side toward center. Tightly roll up to secure filling. Cut in half to serve.

NUTRITION

Amount per serving

Servings: 4

Calories: 339

Fat calories: 121

Percent values: 36% fat, 35% protein, 29% carb

peachy peanut butter pitas

Ingredients

4 pita breads

³/₄ cup crunchy peanut butter

2 fresh peaches, thinly sliced

Step 1: Cut about 3 inches off one edge of pita bread.

Step 2: Spread a thin layer of peanut butter on both inside walls.

Step 3: Fill with peaches; warm pita bread slightly.

NUTRITION

Amount per serving

Servings: 4

Calories: 430

Fat calories: 223

Percent values: 52% fat, 15% protein, 33% carb

mini chickpea cakes

Ingredients

1 can (15 ounces) chickpeas, rinsed and drained

1 cup shredded carrots

$\frac{1}{3}$ cup seasoned dry bread crumbs

$\frac{1}{4}$ cup creamy Italian salad dressing

1 egg

Step 1: Preheat oven to 375 degrees. Spray baking sheet with nonstick cooking spray.

Step 2: Mash chickpeas coarsely in medium bowl with a potato masher. Stir in carrots, bread crumbs, salad dressing, and egg. Mix well.

Step 3: Use a tablespoon to scoop chickpea mixture; form each scoop into small cake or patty shape. Place on prepared baking sheet.

Step 4: Bake 15 to 18 minutes, turning halfway through baking time, until chickpea cakes are lightly browned on both sides. Serve warm with additional salad dressing for dipping.

NUTRITION
Amount per serving
Servings: 24
Calories: 35
Fat calories: 6
Percent values: 17% fat, 16% protein, 67% carb

spinach rice salad

Ingredients

6 cups cooked rice

1 cup coarsely chopped spinach leaves

1 cup crumbled feta cheese

1¼ cups thinly sliced fresh mushrooms

½ cup honey mustard salad dressing

Step 1: Toss all ingredients in a large bowl until combined. Serve.

NUTRITION

Amount per serving

Servings: 6

Calories: 297

Fat calories: 33

Percent values: 11% fat, 15% protein, 74% carb

CHILI BLANCO

Ingredients

$\frac{1}{2}$ pound diced turkey breast

1 tablespoon vegetable oil

$\frac{1}{2}$ cup diced celery

$\frac{1}{2}$ cup chili peppers

$\frac{1}{2}$ cup chopped onions

2 cups water

1 can (16 ounces) small white beans or white kidney beans, drained

1 cup seeded and diced tomatoes

1 cup seeded and diced zucchini

$\frac{1}{2}$ teaspoon salt

$\frac{1}{2}$ teaspoon ground cumin

$\frac{1}{8}$ teaspoon black pepper

$\frac{1}{8}$ teaspoon cayenne pepper

Step 1: Brown turkey in oil in medium saucepan; drain excess drippings. Add celery, chili, and onion; cook until tender.

Step 2: Add remaining ingredients; mix well.

Step 3: Bring mixture to a boil, reduce heat, and simmer 30 minutes or until flavors are blended. Serve with tortillas and condiments—shredded low-fat cheese, salsa, chopped onion, and diced tomato.

NUTRITION
Amount per serving
Servings: 4
Calories: 347
Fat calories: 58
Percent values: 17% fat, 17% protein, 66% carb

Pizza in a Pita

Ingredients
1 whole wheat pita
$^1/_4$ cup grated mozzarella cheese
2 tablespoons pizza sauce
Pepperoni, broccoli, or other toppings

Step 1: Preheat oven to 350 degrees.

Step 2: Split pita bread halfway around the edge; spoon in the cheese, pizza sauce, and any toppings desired.

Step 3: Wrap pita in aluminum foil. Bake for 7 to 10 minutes or until cheese melts.

*Note: Nutritional values are based on a pizza with pepperoni only as the topping.

NUTRITION
Amount per serving
Servings: 1
Calories: 352
Fat calories: 189
Percent values: 54% fat, 16% protein, 30% carb

peanut spinach balls

Ingredients

2 (10-ounce) packages frozen chopped spinach

1 small onion, finely chopped

2 cups dry bread stuffing

$^1/_4$ cup grated Parmesan cheese

4 eggs, well beaten

$^3/_4$ cup butter, melted

$^1/_2$ teaspoon ground thyme

$^1/_4$ teaspoon garlic powder

$^1/_4$ teaspoon salt

$^1/_4$ teaspoon black pepper

1 cup finely chopped roasted peanuts

Step 1: Cook spinach according to package directions or until tender. Drain well. Mix spinach with remaining ingredients, except peanuts, and chill.

Step 2: Shape into 1-inch balls; roll each ball in peanuts. (This recipe can be made ahead and frozen. Freeze, uncooked, on a tray and then transfer to a tightly closed container. Remove the number needed from freezer when ready to cook.)

Step 3: Preheat oven to 350 degrees. Bake for 15 minutes or until lightly browned.

NUTRITION
Amount per serving
Servings: 24
Calories: 81
Fat calories: 47
Percent values: 58% fat, 17% protein, 15% carb

Grilled Eggplant Salad

Ingredients

2 tablespoons extra virgin olive oil

2 teaspoons oregano leaves

2 eggplants cut lengthwise into $\frac{1}{2}$-inch-thick slices

Nonstick cooking spray

$\frac{1}{2}$ teaspoon salt

$\frac{1}{4}$ teaspoon coarsely ground pepper

1 ounce ricotta or feta cheese

2 plum tomatoes cut into $\frac{1}{2}$-inch dice

Lemon wedges

Step 1: Prepare grill to medium-high heat.

Step 2: In small saucepan, heat oil over medium heat until hot, remove from heat; add oregano. Let steep until ready to serve.

Step 3: Lightly spray both sides of eggplant slices with nonstick cooking spray; sprinkle with salt and pepper. Place eggplant on hot grill rack. Cover grill and cook eggplant 7 to 10 minutes or until tender and browned, turning over once.

Step 4: Transfer eggplant to platter; drizzle with oregano oil, and top with ricotta and tomatoes. Serve with lemon wedges.

NUTRITION

Amount per serving

Servings: 8

Calories: 85

Fat calories: 36

Percent values: 42% fat, 10% protein, 48% carb

CLUB TURKEY PASTA SALAD

Ingredients

Dressing

³/₄ cup light mayo

1 teaspoon sugar

¹/₈ teaspoon pepper

2 tablespoons milk

2 tablespoons white wine vinegar

2 teaspoons Dijon mustard

Salad

6 ounces uncooked pasta nuggets (rigatore)

6 slices bacon

2 cups shredded lettuce

6 ounces turkey breast, cubed

3 ounces Monterey Jack cheese blend, cubed

8 cherry tomatoes

1 ripe avocado, peeled, pitted, and cubed

Step 1: In small bowl, combine all dressing ingredients; mix well. Refrigerate while cooking pasta.

Step 2: Cook pasta to desired doneness as directed on package. Drain; rinse with cold water to cool. Drain well.

Step 3: Cook bacon until crisp. Drain on paper towel. Crumble bacon.

Step 4: In large bowl, combine cooked pasta nuggets, bacon, and all remaining salad ingredients. Pour dressing over salad; toss gently to coat.

NUTRITION
Amount per serving
Servings: 6
Calories: 322
Fat calories: 176
Percent values: 58% fat, 19% protein, 23% carb

Chapter 11

DInner:
DInner DeLIGHTS

WHAT'S THE DeaL with dinner? Take-out, opening a can or microwave fare, and good old-fashioned home cooking are options we bring to our tables. Dinner serves more than food. It's a family's time together, sharing stories along with a nutritious meal. Make it and they will come.

Why are family meals so powerful? For one, they give parents an opportunity to model good eating habits and to show kids what a "normal" meal might look like (unlike the French fries/hot dog/soft drink combo they might otherwise choose). It's one of the few opportunities families have to be together as a group, sharing in conversation. As people, we all have a biological need to eat and a social need to eat together. This need for connection doesn't end when kids enter the "My parents are so lame" teen years, either. You can expect some initial rebellion or awkwardness if your family is not used to regular dinners together. But, like exercise, the benefits will accrue only if you stick with it.

Dinner also provides us with one more chance to get in the balanced fuel we need each day. If you missed breakfast and didn't prepare a healthy lunch, chances are you haven't met your energy needs for the day. Don't worry, there's still dinner. Dinner can balance the scales and fill in the gaps left from unhealthy eating habits earlier in the day. Since it is the last meal of the day, we rely on it to get us through the night and to the breakfast table. And as with a car, the night before a trip you fill the gas tank and make sure everything is in working order before heading out to the highway the next morning.

There are times when you're short on time or energy, and you choose to eat out or pick up a deli chicken already prepared to bring home. Remember to save the leftovers for tomorrow's lunches. Other times you'll opt to cook. When you do cook, double the main course recipe and freeze the extra portion to serve on a busy evening. To get started, use the following variety of dinner recipes that are sure to satisfy. Bon appétit!

Barbecue Turkey Sloppy Joes

PREP TIME: 30 MINUTES

Ingredients

2 pounds ground turkey

30 ounces tomato sauce

6 ounces tomato paste

$\frac{1}{2}$ cup brown sugar

$\frac{1}{3}$ cup red wine vinegar

2 tablespoons Worcestershire

2 tablespoons hickory smoke flavor

$\frac{1}{4}$ teaspoon salt

$\frac{1}{4}$ teaspoon pepper

Step 1: In a large skillet, cook turkey over medium heat until lightly browned and crumbly (7 minutes). Drain off extra liquid.

Step 2: Transfer to a 4-quart slow cooker. Stir in sauce, paste, brown sugar, vinegar, Worcestershire, 1 T hickory flavoring, salt, and pepper.

Step 3: Cover and cook on low 6 hours. Stir in remaining hickory flavoring. Serve warm.

NUTRITION

Amount per serving

Servings: 8

Calories: 352

Fat calories: 98

Percent values: 28% fat, 35% protein, 37% carb

peanut Ginger pasta salad

PREP TIME: 40 MINUTES

Ingredients

4 ounces bow-tie pasta

1 cup mushrooms

1 cup squash

2 carrots, sliced

1 cucumber, sliced

$^3/_4$ cup green beans

2 plum tomatoes

$^3/_4$ cup ginger dressing (see step 1)

Step 1: Ginger dressing: Mix $^1/_2$ cup coconut milk, $^1/_4$ cup oil, 2 tablespoons squash, and 2 tablespoons white vinegar. Add 1 packet Thai Spicy Peanut salad dressing mix and 1 tablespoon grated ginger. Blend for 2 minutes.

Step 2: Cook pasta; rinse with cold water. Drain and put into mixing bowl.

Step 3: Add all veggies cut and sliced, except tomatoes.

Step 4: Add ginger dressing.

Step 5: Add tomatoes and served chilled.

NUTRITION
Amount per serving
Servings: 4
Calories: 282
Fat calories: 147
Percent values: 52% fat, 8% protein, 40% carb

CHICKEN NUGGETS

Ingredients

1 egg

2 tablespoons milk

3½ cups corn flakes

1 pound boneless, skinless chicken breasts, cut into nugget-size
pieces

¼ cup barbecue sauce, ketchup, or ranch dressing for dipping sauce

Step 1: Preheat oven to 400 degrees.

Step 2: Whisk the egg and milk together in a small mixing bowl.

Step 3: Place cornflakes in a plastic bag; crush.

Step 4: Dip chicken pieces in egg mixture, and then shake in the
plastic bag with cornflakes to coat.

Step 5: Place coated chicken on a baking sheet. Bake for 15 minutes. Serve with one or all the dipping sauces.

NUTRITION
Amount per serving
Servings: 6
Calories: 463
Fat calories: 206
Percent values: 44% fat, 30% protein, 26% carb

Tuna Burgers

Ingredients

1 (12-ounce) can tuna, drained and flaked

1 1/2 cups bread crumbs

1 cup shredded cheddar cheese

1 egg, lightly beaten

1/2 cup nonfat peppercorn ranch salad dressing

1/4 cup sliced green onion

1 tablespoon olive oil

Step 1: In a medium bowl, combine tuna, 3/4 cup bread crumbs, cheese, egg, salad dressing, and onion.

Step 2: Form six patties; coat each side with remaining 3/4 cup bread crumbs.

Step 3: Heat oil in nonstick skillet over medium heat.

Step 4: Cook patties 3 to 5 minutes on each side until golden brown.

NUTRITION
Amount per serving
Servings: 6
Calories: 308
Fat calories: 99
Percent values: 32% fat, 34% protein, 34% carb

cheese spinach noodles

Ingredients

8 ounces egg noodles

1 (10-ounce) package frozen chopped spinach, thawed and drained

$\frac{1}{2}$ teaspoon dried basil

1 tablespoon dried parsley flakes

1 cup fat-free cottage cheese

$\frac{1}{4}$ teaspoon salt

2 tablespoons Parmesan cheese

Step 1: Cook noodles according to package directions.

Step 2: While noodles are cooking, cook spinach in a skillet for 5 minutes.

Step 3: Add basil, parsley, cottage cheese, and salt to spinach. Cook 3 more minutes, or until heated.

Step 4: Drain noodles and toss in large serving bowl with the spinach mixture. Top with Parmesan cheese. Serve.

NUTRITION
Amount per serving
Servings: 6
Calories: 104
Fat calories: 14
Percent values: 13% fat, 42% protein, 45% carb

sesame shrimp and asparagus

PREP TIME: 25 MINUTES

Ingredients

1 cup jasmine rice

$1/_8$ teaspoon salt

4 teaspoons olive oil

$1^1/_2$ teaspoons sesame oil

$1/_4$ cup soy sauce

2 pounds asparagus, trimmed

2 teaspoons seasoned rice vinegar

1 large green onion

1 pound large shrimp

$1/_8$ teaspoon crushed red pepper

Step 1: Preheat oven to 450 degrees. Prepare rice as label directs.

Step 2: Combine salt, 2 teaspoons olive oil, and 1 teaspoon sesame oil in a cup. Roast asparagus in pan with oil mixture for 10 to 12 minutes, until tender.

Step 3: In a small bowl, whisk soy sauce, vinegar, green onion, and remaining $1/_2$ teaspoon sesame oil; set aside. Shell and devein shrimp.

Step 4: In a nonstick 12-inch skillet, heat 2 teaspoons olive oil over medium heat until very hot. Add shrimp; sprinkle with red pepper and cook 3 minutes, stirring frequently.

Step 5: Arrange shrimp, asparagus, and rice on four plates; drizzle with dressing. Serve.

NUTRITION
Amount per serving
Servings: 4
Calories: 370
Fat calories: 80
Percent values: 22% fat, 31% protein, 47% carb

SPICED PORK TENDERLOINS

Ingredients

Salsa

2 ripe mangoes, peeled and chopped

2 medium kiwi, peeled and chopped

2 tablespoons seasoned rice vinegar

1 tablespoon grated peeled fresh ginger

1 tablespoon minced fresh cilantro leaves

Tenderloins

2 whole pork tenderloins

3 tablespoons flour

1 teaspoon salt

1 teaspoon ground cumin

1 teaspoon ground coriander

$\frac{1}{2}$ teaspoon ground cinnamon

$\frac{1}{2}$ teaspoon ground pepper

Step 1: Prepare mango salsa: In medium bowl, combine mangoes, kiwi fruit, vinegar, ginger, cilantro. Cover and refrigerate up to 4 hours.

Step 2: Prepare grill for grilling over medium heat.

Step 3: Meanwhile, cut each pork tenderloin lengthwise almost in half, being careful not to cut all the way through. Open and spread flat. Place each tenderloin between two sheets of plastic wrap; with meat mallet, pound to $\frac{1}{4}$-inch thickness. Cut each tenderloin into four pieces.

Step 4: On waxed paper, mix flour, salt, cumin, coriander, cinnamon, and pepper. Add pork to spice mixture and turn to coat evenly.

Step 5: Place pork on hot grill rack. Cover and cook pork 5 to 6 minutes or until lightly browned on both sides, turning pork over once. Spoon mango salsa over each tenderloin. Serve warm.

NUTRITION

Amount per serving

Servings: 8

Calories: 215

Fat calories: 54

Percent values: 24% fat, 30% protein, 46% carb

---

carrot risotto

Ingredients

1 (12-ounce) can carrot juice

1 (14.5-ounce) can chicken or vegetable broth (1¾ cups)

½ cup dry white wine

1 tablespoon olive oil

2 cups shredded carrots

½ small onion, finely chopped

2 cups arborio rice (Italian)

⅓ cup grated Parmesan cheese

¾ teaspoon salt

¼ teaspoon ground black pepper

2 tablespoons chopped mint or parsley

Step 1: In a covered 2-quart saucepan, heat carrot juice, broth, wine, and 1¼ cups water to boiling over high heat.

Step 2: In a 3½-quart microwave-safe casserole dish, combine oil, carrots, and onion. Cook, uncovered, in microwave oven on high for 2 minutes or until onion softens. Add rice and stir to coat. Cook on high 1 minute.

Step 3: Stir hot liquid into rice mixture. Cover casserole dish with lid or vented plastic wrap and cook on medium (50 percent power) for 15 to 20 minutes or until most of the liquid is absorbed and rice is tender but still firm. Stir in Parmesan, salt, and pepper. Sprinkle top with mint or parsley if desired.

NUTRITION

Amount per serving

Servings: 4

Calories: 565

Fat calories: 65

Percent values: 13% fat, 19% protein, 68% carb

Tangy Citrus Chicken

Ingredients

8 boneless, skinless chicken breasts

1 (6-ounce) can frozen lemonade concentrate, thawed

1/2 cup honey

1 teaspoon rubbed sage

1/2 teaspoon ground mustard

1/2 teaspoon dried thyme

1/2 teaspoon lemon juice

Step 1: Preheat oven to 350 degrees. Place chicken breasts in a 13 × 9 × 2 baking dish coated with nonstick cooking spray.

Step 2: In a small bowl, combine remaining ingredients; mix well.

Step 3: Pour half the sauce over chicken. Bake uncovered for 20 minutes.

Step 4: Turn chicken; pour remaining sauce on top. Bake 15 to 20 minutes longer or until meat juices run clear.

NUTRITION
Amount per serving
Servings: 8
Calories: 268
Fat calories: 36
Percent values: 13% fat, 67% protein, 20% carb

Chapter 12

snacks: morninG GLories
anD Brain Breaks

WHAT IS "smarT snackinG"? Kids need snacks, or "mini-meals," to help them get enough calories (energy) throughout the day and help fill nutrient gaps. Choosing healthy foods that add nutrients to their diets is essential and smart snacking. Combine snacks from at least two food groups, like a protein and a carbohydrate, to pack more nutrients into your child's diet. It will be more filling and will tide them over until their next meal. Fresh fruits and vegetables and "go-together" foods such as cereal and milk, peanut butter and celery, or cheese and crackers are ready-to-eat, quick-energy snacks. Adding 1 percent or skim milk to cereal and graham crackers or peanut butter to crackers or fruit is an easy way to add calcium and protein to an otherwise carbohydrate-only snack.

If chosen carefully, snacks can promote good health by supplying nutrients without adding too many calories. Remember to keep snack portions small, and space snacks far enough away from meals so appetites are not spoiled. Next time you or your kids need to refuel, try any of the following quick, healthy snacks.

Fruit Pita

Ingredients

1 whole wheat pita, cut in half

$\frac{1}{2}$ cup fat-free cottage cheese

$\frac{1}{2}$ cup pineapple chunks in juice

Step 1: Toast pita halves.

Step 2: Stuff each pita half with cottage cheese and pineapple.

NUTRITION
Amount per serving
Servings: 2
Calories: 140
Fat calories: 0
Percent values: 0% fat, 26% protein, 74% carb

pretzel kabobs

Ingredients

$1/2$ ounce fat-free pretzel sticks

2 ounces baked lean ham or chicken chunks

1 ounce reduced fat cheese, cut into chunks

Step 1: Allow kids to build their own kabobs by skewering meat and cheese chunks with pretzels.

NUTRITION
Amount per serving
Servings: 1
Calories: 275
Fat calories: 63
Percent values: 23% fat, 44% protein, 33% carb

FruIT KaBOBS

Ingredients

$\frac{1}{2}$ cup fresh strawberries

$\frac{1}{2}$ cup banana

$\frac{1}{2}$ cup grapes

$\frac{1}{2}$ cup pineapple chunks in juice

1 cup fat-free plain yogurt

Step 1: Let kids build their own kabobs by alternating fruit chunks on straws.

Step 2: Dip into yogurt.

NUTRITION

Amount per serving

Servings: 2

Calories: 117

Fat calories: 0

Percent values: 0% fat, 12% protein, 88% carb

Frozen Fruit Pops

Ingredients

¹/₂ cup 100 percent fruit juice

¹/₂ cup pineapple chunks in juice

1 cup fat-free yogurt

2 plastic cups

2 spoons

Step 1: Pour fruit, yogurt, and juice into a blender; blend until smooth.

Step 2: Pour into two small plastic cups and insert spoon; freeze.

NUTRITION
Amount per serving
Servings: 2
Calories: 132
Fat calories: 0
Percent values: 0% fat, 13% protein, 87% carb

veggie bowl

Ingredients

1 green pepper

2 celery stalks, sliced and cut into 4-inch pieces

10 baby carrots

¹/₄ cup fat-free salad dressing of choice

Step 1: Wash vegetables and slice celery.

Step 2: Cut top off pepper; remove seeds from inside to form veggie bowl.

Step 3: Pour salad dressing into halved pepper and stack celery and carrots inside.

NUTRITION

Amount per serving

Servings: 1

Calories: 132

Fat calories: 0

Percent values: 0% fat, 1% protein, 99% carb

Fruit Jell-O

Ingredients

1 package sugar-free, fruit-flavored gelatin of choice
1 cup sliced fresh strawberries
8 tablespoons reduced fat whipped topping

Step 1: Prepare gelatin as directed on package; add fruit.

Step 2: Pour into individual dessert cups and refrigerate until jelled. Top with whipped topping.

NUTRITION
Amount per serving
Servings: 4
Calories: 64
Fat calories: 36
Percent values: 56% fat, 7% protein, 37% carb

ants on a LOG

Ingredients
2 stalks celery
1 tablespoon peanut butter
$\frac{1}{4}$ cup raisins

Step 1: Wash celery stalks and cut into 1-inch pieces (logs).

Step 2: Spread peanut butter on stalks; place raisins in a single-file line in peanut butter (ants).

NUTRITION
Amount per serving
Servings: 1
Calories: 169
Fat calories: 49
Percent values: 29% fat, 14% protein, 57% carb

apple volcanoes

Ingredients

1 medium apple

1 tablespoon reduced fat peanut butter

2 tablespoons raisins

2 tablespoons granola

Step 1: Cut top off apple; remove core.

Step 2: Fill center with peanut butter; sprinkle with granola and raisins.

NUTRITION
Amount per serving
Servings: 1
Calories: 247
Fat calories: 58
Percent values: 23% fat, 9% protein, 68% carb

Butterfly Sandwiches

Ingredients

1 4-ounce boneless, skinless chicken breast half, baked and shredded

4 slices fat-free whole wheat bread

2 tablespoons fat-free ranch dressing

2 4-inch carrot sticks

$^1/_4$ cup raisins

Step 1: In a small mixing bowl, mix chicken and ranch dressing; spread on bread to make a sandwich.

Step 2: Cut sandwich into triangles. Use a carrot stick for the body and raisins for the eyes.

NUTRITION
Amount per serving
Servings: 2
Calories: 295
Fat calories: 23
Percent values: 1% fat, 33% protein, 66% carb

ITALIAN CHICKEN PITAS

Ingredients

1 4-ounce boneless, skinless chicken breast half, baked and cubed

$\frac{1}{2}$ cup reduced fat chunky vegetable spaghetti sauce

1 whole wheat pita, halved and warmed

Step 1: In a bowl, stir together spaghetti sauce and chicken.

Step 2: Heat in microwave until warm, about 1 minute.

Step 3: Spoon mixture into pita bread halves.

NUTRITION
Amount per serving
Servings: 2
Calories: 216
Fat calories: 36
Percent values: 17% fat, 39% protein, 44% carb

Fun Mix

Ingredients

1 cup popcorn

1 cup pretzels

$\frac{1}{2}$ cup raisins

$\frac{1}{2}$ cup chocolate candies

$\frac{1}{2}$ cup dried cranberries

1 cup Trix cereal

Step 1: Mix all ingredients together in a large mixing bowl. Separate into 6 cups. Serve.

NUTRITION

Amount per serving

Servings: 6

Calories: 290

Fat calories: 32

Percent values: 12% fat, 10% protein, 78% carb

Fresh Fruit Pizza

Ingredients

20 ounces cookie dough

8 ounces light cream cheese

$\frac{1}{3}$ cup sugar

1 teaspoon vanilla extract

2 kiwis, peeled and sliced

1 can pineapple chunks

$\frac{1}{4}$ cup raspberries

1 banana

$\frac{1}{4}$ cup apricot jam, melted

Step 1: Press cookie dough onto 14-inch pizza pan. Bake at 350 degrees for 13 minutes until browned.

Step 2: Beat cream cheese, sugar, and vanilla. Spread over cooled cookie.

Step 3: Cut and slice pineapple, kiwi, banana, and raspberries. Arrange fruit overlapping toward the center. Brush with jam.

NUTRITION
Amount per serving
Servings: 8
Calories: 464
Fat calories: 141
Percent values: 29% fat, 6% protein, 65% carb

Fruit Smoothie

Ingredients

1$\frac{1}{2}$ cups milk

2 ripe bananas

1 cup vanilla yogurt

$\frac{1}{4}$ cup honey

1 teaspoon vanilla

$\frac{1}{2}$ teaspoon cinnamon

Dash of nutmeg

5 ice cubes

Step 1: In a blender, combine all ingredients and blend until smooth.

NUTRITION

Amount per serving

Servings: 2

Calories: 270

Fat calories: 21

Percent values: 8% fat, 15% protein, 77% carb

PITA TRIANGLES

Ingredients

3 large whole wheat tortillas

$\frac{1}{4}$ cup sugar

1 tablespoon cinnamon

Creamy dip (see step 5)

Step 1: Cut the large tortillas into six equal triangles per tortilla.

Step 2: Mix the sugar and cinnamon in a small bowl.

Step 3: Lay the triangles in a single layer on a baking sheet; sprinkle them lightly with the cinnamon sugar mixture.

Step 4: Bake at 350 degrees for 15 minutes. Serve warm or room temperature with dip.

Step 5: Prepare creamy dip: Mix together in a small bowl $\frac{1}{2}$ cup cream cheese, $\frac{1}{4}$ cup peanut butter, and 1 tablespoon cinnamon until smooth.

NUTRITION
Amount per serving
Servings: 3
Calories: 146
Fat calories: 27
Percent values: 18% fat, 1% protein, 81% carb

peanutty banana dip

Ingredients

$\frac{1}{2}$ cup sliced banana

$\frac{1}{3}$ cup creamy peanut butter

2 tablespoons fat-free milk

1 tablespoon honey

$\frac{1}{2}$ teaspoon vanilla

$\frac{1}{2}$ teaspoon ground cinnamon

Step 1: Place all ingredients in blender and process until smooth. Serve with celery sticks, apple slices, or pita triangles.

NUTRITION
Amount per serving
Servings: 4
Calories: 99
Fat calories: 54
Percent values: 55% fat, 2% protein, 43% carb

Banana Rolls

Ingredients

1 banana

2 tablespoons peanut butter

$\frac{1}{4}$ cup rice cereal

Step 1: Peel and cut banana in quarters crosswise.

Step 2: Spread with peanut butter.

Step 3: Roll in rice cereal. Serve immediately or chill for later.

NUTRITION

Amount per serving

Servings: 2

Calories: 193

Fat calories: 73

Percent values: 38% fat, 12% protein, 50% carb

Tree snacks

Ingredients

2 carrots cut into strips

1 cup broccoli

1 cup cauliflower

Low-fat ranch dressing

Step 1: Wash and cut up vegetables.

Step 2: Put carrots on a plate vertically (tree trunk). Put broccoli and cauliflower florets at the top of the carrot sticks (tree top).

Step 3: Dip vegetables in the ranch dressing and enjoy!

NUTRITION

Amount per serving

Servings: 4

Calories: 56

Fat calories: 16

Percent values: 29% fat, 7% protein, 64% carb

STUFFED APPLE RINGS

Ingredients

1/3 cup dried cranberries

1/4 cup pecan pieces

2 tablespoons butter, softened

1 tablespoon packed brown sugar

1 teaspoon ground cinnamon

1/2 teaspoon vanilla

2 medium apples

Step 1: Preheat oven to 425 degrees. Line a baking sheet with foil; set aside.

Step 2: In a medium bowl, mix cranberries, pecans, butter, sugar, cinnamon, and vanilla. Stir until combined.

Step 3: Slice ends off apples. Core and slice each apple into four round slices, to yield eight rings total.

Step 4: Coat baking sheet with cooking spray and arrange apple slices in a single layer on baking sheet. Spoon equal amounts of cranberry mixture in the center of each apple slice.

Step 5: Bake for 10 minutes or until apples are tender. Serve warm or room temperature.

NUTRITION
Amount per serving
Servings: 4
Calories: 140
Fat calories: 71
Percent values: 51% fat, 2% protein, 47% carb

SPICY snakes

Ingredients

1 (8-ounce) package refrigerated crescent rolls
1 peach cut into 8 slices
16 raisins
Dash ground cinnamon

Step 1: Separate rolls and stretch lightly. Place peach slice on wide end and roll up to resemble a snake.

Step 2: Place on baking sheet. Press in two raisin "eyes" and sprinkle lightly with cinnamon.

Step 3: Bake according to package directions or until golden brown.

NUTRITION
Amount per serving
Servings: 8
Calories: 144
Fat calories: 36
Percent values: 25% fat, 1% protein, 74% carb

Honey Bran Squares

Ingredients

$\frac{1}{4}$ cup honey

$\frac{1}{4}$ cup butter

4 cups miniature marshmallows

6 cups favorite bran cereal

1 cup peanuts

Step 1: Blend honey and butter in large saucepan; stir in marshmallows.

Step 2: Cook and stir over medium-high heat until marshmallows are melted.

Step 3: Mix together cereal and nuts; stir in marshmallow mixture until well coated.

Step 4: Press into lightly greased 13 × 9 × 2 inch pan. Cut into squares.

NUTRITION

Amount per serving

Servings: 24

Calories: 135

Fat calories: 45

Percent values: 34% fat, 9% protein, 57% carb

FIVE-FRUIT SALAD

Ingredients

1 (15-ounce) can pineapple chunks in juice
1 (15-ounce) can mandarin orange segments
1 (8-ounce) jar maraschino cherries, pitted
1 cup light sour cream
1 (4-ounce) package instant vanilla pudding mix

Step 1: Drain pineapple chunks, cherries, and mandarin orange segments. Mix together in a large bowl.

Step 2: In a separate bowl, mix together sour cream and instant vanilla pudding mix.

Step 3: Add fruit mixture to cream mixture; stir gently. Chill for 2 hours. Serve.

NUTRITION
Amount per serving
Servings: 8
Calories: 150
Fat calories: 32
Percent values: 20% fat, 5% protein, 75% carb

more Fruit kabobs

Ingredients

$\frac{1}{2}$ cup strawberries

$\frac{1}{2}$ medium cantaloupe

1 banana

2 kiwis or any other in season fruit

Skewers, toothpicks, or plastic straws*

Step 1: Cut up fruits into chunks.

Step 2: Place on skewers, toothpicks, or plastic straws.

*Note: Fruit kabobs on straws are a fun way to encourage water drinking. Have children stir their straw with the fruits attached into the water cup for "flavor."

NUTRITION
Amount per serving
Servings: 2
Calories: 158
Fat calories: 18
Percent values: 11% fat, 6% protein, 83% carb

snack mix

Ingredients

2 cups dried cereal (Chex, Cheerios, corn flakes)

1 cup raisins

1 cup nuts

1 cup dates or other dried fruit

Step 1: Pour all ingredients into a large mixing bowl.

Step 2: Cover and shake until all ingredients are mixed.

NUTRITION
Amount per serving
Servings: 4
Calories: 140
Fat calories: 63
Percent values: 45% fat, 11% protein, 44% carb

Frozen Apple Fruit Cup

PREP TIME: 60 MINUTES

Ingredients

1 cup applesauce

1 (10–ounce) package frozen strawberries, thawed

1 (11-ounce) can mandarin orange segments, drained

1 cup seedless grapes

2 tablespoons orange juice concentrate

Step 1: In a medium bowl, combine all ingredients.

Step 2: Spoon fruit mixture into individual dishes or paper cups.

Step 3: Freeze until firm. Remove from freezer about 30 minutes before serving.

NUTRITION
Amount per serving
Servings: 4
Calories: 150
Fat calories: 15
Percent values: 10% fat, 5% protein, 85% carb

Banana pops

Ingredients

1 package instant banana pudding

2 cups skim milk

1 banana, cut into pieces

Step 1: Combine pudding mix and milk.

Step 2: Add cut banana into pudding and blend evenly.

Step 3: Spoon enough pudding/bananas into ice-pop cups to cover bottom.

Freeze until set.

NUTRITION
Amount per serving
Servings: 4
Calories: 181
Fat calories: 40
Percent values: 22% fat, 10% protein, 68% carb

YOGURT PARFAIT

Ingredients

$\frac{1}{4}$ cup Grape Nuts

16-ounce carton lemon or vanilla yogurt

$\frac{1}{4}$ cup fruit of choice

Step 1: Sprinkle Grape Nuts at the bottom of a cup.

Step 2: Add a spoonful of yogurt. Add fruit and top with more yogurt.

Step 3: Sprinkle Grape Nuts on top. Chill for 30 minutes.

NUTRITION
Amount per serving
Servings: 2
Calories: 160
Fat calories: 43
Percent values: 27% fat, 25% protein, 48% carb

carrot raisin rounds

Ingredients

1 carrot, grated

$\frac{1}{4}$ cup raisins

$\frac{1}{4}$ cup walnuts

2 tablespoons mayonnaise

2 tablespoons plain yogurt

1 teaspoon lemon juice

4 slices raisin English muffins

Step 1: Clean carrot and shred into small pieces.

Step 2: Mix all ingredients except bread. Spread on English muffin halves.

NUTRITION

Amount per serving

Servings: 4

Calories: 289

Fat calories: 103

Percent values: 36% fat, 11% protein, 53% carb

GRAHAM CRACKER FACE-UPS

Ingredients

1 graham cracker

1 tablespoon peanut butter

Add-ons: $\frac{1}{4}$ banana, sliced, 2 tablespoons applesauce,
or 2 tablespoons crushed pineapple

Sprinkle-ons: 1 teaspoon raisins, sunflower seeds, rice cereal,
coconut, or granola

Step 1: Break graham cracker into two squares. Spread peanut butter on cracker.

Step 2: Select one add-on to spread on top of the peanut butter.

Step 3: Select and sprinkle one or more of the sprinkle-ons on top.

NUTRITION
Amount per serving
Servings: 1
Calories: 236
Fat calories: 90
Percent values: 38% fat, 10% protein, 52% carb

SMOOTHIE POPS

Ingredients

5 strawberries
1 medium banana
4 ice cubes
1 cup strawberry yogurt
$\frac{1}{2}$ cup milk
$\frac{1}{2}$ cup fruit juice

Step 1: Mix all ingredients in a blender until smooth. Pour into 3-ounce paper cups, cover with plastic wrap, and insert wooden sticks. Freeze for at least 5 hours.

NUTRITION
Amount per serving
Servings: 12
Calories: 50
Fat calories: 9
Percent values: 18% fat, 11% protein, 71% carb

easy applesauce muffins

Ingredients

6 tablespoons butter

1 1/2 cups flour

1 teaspoon baking powder

1/2 teaspoon baking soda

1 teaspoon cinnamon

1/2 teaspoon salt

2 eggs

2/3 cup brown sugar

1 1/2 cups chunky applesauce

Step 1: Heat oven to 375 degrees. Line a 12-cup muffin pan with baking cups.

Step 2: In a small microwave-safe bowl, melt butter; set aside.

Step 3: Sift together flour, baking powder, baking soda, cinnamon, and salt into a large mixing bowl.

Step 4: In another large bowl, whisk together eggs and brown sugar. Stir in applesauce and melted butter until mixture is smooth.

Step 5: Pour the apple mixture over the flour mixture. Mix until completely blended.

Step 6: Fill the baking cups about two-thirds full with batter. Bake for 20 minutes or until light brown.

NUTRITION
Amount per serving
Servings: 12
Calories: 190
Fat calories: 64
Percent values: 34% fat, <1% protein, 65% carb

Appendix A

TO FIND OUT more
CHAPTER BY CHAPTER

THE FOLLOWING LISTS include recommended readings from each chapter, as well as references used in the writing of this book. The organizations listed will assist you in finding further information on the subject matter from each chapter as needed. Please know these are only a few of many sources of information on all the different subjects we touch on in this book dealing with children, nutrition, behavior, and performance.

CHAPTER 1: FEED THE BODY AND THE MIND

The Amazing Brain by Robert Ornstein and Richard F. Thompson. Boston: Houghton Mifflin, 1984.

The Brain by Richard Restak. New York: Bantam, 1984.

The Brain Food Diet for Children by Ralph E. Minear. New York: Bobbs-Merrill, 1983.

Can Your Child Read? Is He Hyperactive? by William G. Crook. Jackson, TN: Professional Books, 1978.

From Classroom to Cafeteria: A Nutrition Guide for Teachers and Managers by Sara Sloan. Atlanta: Nutra Program, 1978.

The Conscious Brain by Steven Ross. New York: Knopf, 1973.

Mind, Mood, and Medicine by Paul H. Wneder and Donald F. Klein. New York: Farrar, Straus, & Giroux, 1981.

Nutrition and Mental Function by G. Serban, editor. New York: Plenum, 1975.

Nutrition and Your Mind by George Watson. New York: Harper & Row, 1974.

Overcoming Learning Disabilities by Martin Baren, Robert Leibl, and Lendon Smith. Reston, VA: Reston, 1978.

Amazing Amino Acids by William H. Lee. New Canaan, CT: Pivot/Keats, 1984.

Body, Mind, and the B-Vitamins by Ruth Adams and Frank Murray. New York: Larchmont, 1979.

The Book of Vitamin Therapy by Harold Rosenburg and A. N. Feldzaman. New York: Berkley Books, 1975.

The Brain Chemistry Diet by Michael Lesser, M.D. New York: Putnam's, 2002.

Mega Nutrients for Your Nerves by H. L. Newbold. New York: Wydon, 1975.

The Pediatrics Guide to Drug and Vitamins by Edward R. Brace. New York: Delacorte/Stonesong, 1982.

Trace Minerals by Erwin DiCyan. New Canaan, CT: Keats, 1984.

Vitamin Bible for Your Kids by Earl Mindell. New York: Bantam, 1982.

The Vitamin Robbers by Earl Mindell and William H. Lee. New Canaan, CT: Keats, 1983.

Vitamins and You by Robert J. Benowicz. New York: Berkley Books, 1981.

Organizations/Websites

American Dietetic Association: www.eatright.org

American Heart Association: www.americanheart.org

Centers for Disease Control: www.cdc.gov

International Food Information Council: www.ific.org

CHAPTERS 3 TO 7:
GROWING BODIES/GROWING MINDS

The following resources are from books and websites available on each topic. There are thousands of resources in the field of nutrition and brain connections, far too many to mention here. However, those listed are selected for their excellence, readability, and availability. They are some of the sources for this book.

ADHD

Child Development and Personality by Paul H. Mussen, John J. Conger, and Jerome Kagan. New York: Harper & Row, 1969.

How to Improve Your Child's Behavior through Diet by Laura J. Stevens and Rosemary B. Stoner. New York: Doubleday, 1979.

Improving Your Child's Behavior Chemistry by Lendon Smith. Englewood Cliffs, NJ: Prentice Hall, 1974.

Nutrition and Your Child's Behavior by Hugh Powers and James Pressley. New York: St. Martin's, 1978.

Nutrition, Development and Social Behavior. Washington, DC: U.S. Government Printing Office, 1973.

Something's Wrong with My Child by Milton Brutten, Sylvia O. Richardson, and Charles Mangel. New York: Harcourt Brace Jovanovich, 1973.

Why Is Your Child Hyperactive? by Ben F. Feingold. New York: Wallaby/Simon & Schuster, 1977.

Organization/Website

National Institute of Child Health and Human Development (part of the National Institutes of Health): www.nih.gov/nichd

Allergies

Allergies and the Hyperactive Child by Doris J. Rapp. New York: Cornerstone/ Simon & Schuster, 1981.

Allergy, Brains, and Children Coping by Ray C. Wunderlich. St. Petersburg, FL: Johnny-Reads, 1973.

Are You Allergic? by William G. Crook. Jackson, TN: Professional Books, 1978.

Infant and Child Feeding by J. T. Bond, editor. New York: Academic Press, 1981.

Sugar Blues by Willam Duffy. New York: Warner Books, 1975.

Understanding Food Allergy by the American Academy of Allergy & Immunology and International Food Information Council Foundation. Informative pamphlet; (800) 822-2762.

Organizations/Websites

Allergy Gear: www.allergygear.com

Allergy Relief Store: www.onlineallergyrelief.com

American Academy of Allergy Asthma and Immunology: www.aaai.org

Food Allergy Network: www.foodallergy.org

International Food Information Council Foundation: www.ific.org

Johns Hopkins Children's Center: www.hopkinschildrens.org

Nemours Foundation: www.kidshealth.org

Athletes

Child's Body by the Diagram Group. New York: Wallaby/Simon & Schuster, 1977.

The Healing Factor by Irwin Stone. New York: Grosset & Dunlap, 1974.

The Pediatric Guide to Drugs and Vitamins by Edward R. Brace. New York: Delacorte/Stonesong, 1982.

Supernutrition by Richard J. Passwater. New York: Dial, 1975.

Organizations/Websites

American Academy of Pediatrics: www.aap.org

American College of Sports Medicine: www.acsm.org

Child and Adolescent Nutrition and Health: www.ificinfo.health.org

Physical Activity and Nutrition Unit: www.eatsmartmovemore.com

Diabetes

Feed Your Kids Right by Lendon Smith. New York: Dell, 1979.

A Guide to Nutra Lunches and Natural Foods by Sara Sloan. Atlanta: Nutra Program, 1977.

Infant and Child Feeding by J. T. Bond, editor. New York: Academic Press, 1981.

Pediatric Nutrition Handbook by the American Academy of Pediatrics. Elk Grove Village, IL: American Academy of Pediatrics, 1993.

The Total Nutrition Guide for Mother and Baby by Alice White. New York: Ballantine/ Random House, 1983.

Organizations/Websites

Child and Adolescent Nutrition and Health: www.ificinfo.health.org

Food Nutrition Information Center: www.nal.usda.gov

Eating Disorders

Body, Mind, and the B-Vitamins by Ruth Adams and Frank Murray. New York: Larchmont, 1979.

The Broken Brain by Nancy C. Andreason. New York: Harper & Row, 1984.

Diet and Disease by E. Cheraskin, W. M. Ringsdorf, and J. W. Clark. New Canaan, CT: Keats, 1978.

The Food Depression Connection by June Roth. Chicago: Contemporary Books, 1978.

Organizations/Websites

American Dietetic Association: www.eatright.org

Centers for Disease Control: www.cdc.gov

Obesity

Diet and Disease by E. Cheraskin, W. M. Ringsdorf, and J. W. Clark. New Canaan, CT: Keats, 1978.

Foods for Healthy Kids by Lendon Smith. New York: McGraw-Hill, 1981.

Healthy Living in an Unhealthy World by Edward J. Calabrese and Michael W. Dorsey. New York: Simon & Schuster, 1984.

The Nutrition Business by John Yudkin. New York: St. Martin's, 1975.

Parent's Guide to Nutrition by Boston Children's Hospital. Boston: Addison-Wesley, 1986.

Organizations/Websites

American Academy of Pediatrics: www.aap.org

North Carolina Healthy Weight in Children Initiative: www.nutritionnc.com

Puberty/Hormones

"Diet in Mid-puberty and Sedentary Activity in Pre-puberty Predict Peak Bone Mass" by M.-C. Wang et al., *American Journal of Clinical Nutrition*, February 2003.

"Nutrition in the Adolescent" by Richard Wahl, *Pediatric Annals*, February 1999.

"Nutrition for Youth" by R. Venkdeswaran, *Clinical Family Practice*, December 2000.

CHAPTER 8: CHALLENGES TO FEEDING OUR KIDS RIGHT

American Dietetic Association's Guide to Healthy Eating for Kids. New York: Wiley, 2002.

The Debt Diet by Ellie Kay. Minneapolis: Bethany House, 2005.

Dietary Guidelines for Americans. www.health.gov/dietaryguidelines.

Healthy Habits for Healthy Kids: A Nutrition and Activity Guide for Parents. www.wellpoint.com/commitments/healthy_parenting.asp#1.

Misery Meals by Jonni McCoy. Minneapolis: Bethany House, 2002.

Poverty: Social Conscience in the Progressive Era by Robert Hunter. New York: Harper & Row, 1965.

Organizations/Websites

Dole 5 a Day: www.dole5aday.com

The Dollar Stretcher: www.stretcher.com

Food, Fun and Facts: www.foodfunandfacts.com

Food Research and Action Center: www.frac.org

Keep Kids Healthy.com (a pediatrician's guide to your children's health and safety): www.keepkidshealthy.com

Kids Daily Food Planner: www.quakeroatmeal.com/partnersnutrition

Living a Better Life—Grocery Saving Tips: www.grocerysavingtips.com

National School Lunch Program: www.fns.usda.gov/cnd/lunch

Nutrition.gov: www.nutrition.gov

School Nutrition Association: www.asfsa.org

Appendix B

sample meal plans

THE FOLLOWING meal plans are only suggestions to get you started on planning a variety of healthy, nutrient-filled meals and snacks to help children achieve success every day at school or home. Seven different meal suggestions are provided for breakfast (eye openers), midmorning snack (morning glories), lunch (lunch bunch), afternoon snack (brain breaks), and dinner (dinner delights). This is to provide you with a full week's worth of menus. Pick one meal or snack from each category for a single day's diet.

The menu plans are further divided into age groups. These age groups correspond directly to the ages discussed in Part II of this book. An asterisk (*) indicates that the recipe may be found in this book.

chapter 3: menus for 1- to 3-year-olds

While a baby is in the womb to when children are very young, the brain grows more rapidly than at any other stage of child development. Brain-building nutrients come from fat. The amount of fat in the diet is important. However, the type of fat is critical. Omega-3 fatty acids found in fish and flax oil and DHA fatty acids are excellent sources of brain-building fats. Adding 2 teaspoons of flax oil to smoothies or juice, and mixing tuna or salmon with macaroni are easy ways to get an early start in adding the important brain-building nutrients into the diet of a very young child.

The following meal plan suggestions are geared toward young children and their age-appropriate needs. There are many other meals one can use. The following are just a few meals to get you started feeding your child smart. In addition, while making new meal plans, keep in mind the need for brain-building fats, and be sure to include the appropriate aforementioned fatty acids.

BREAKFAST

- Oatmeal, milk, ½ cut banana
- Cheese grits, ½ cup applesauce
- On-the-Run Smoothie,* 1 wheat English muffin
- Whole wheat toast with cream cheese and sliced peaches
- 1 egg scrambled with low-fat cheese, ½ cup cut and peeled apples
- Whole wheat buttermilk pancakes, milk, ½ cup blueberries
- Applesauce Muffins,* ½ cup plain yogurt with favorite berries mixed in

MORNING GLORIES

- Low-fat mozzarella cheese stick, ½ cup cut grapes
- Graham cracker spread with 1 tablespoon peanut butter
- ½ cup cut-up fruit of choice, ½ cup vanilla yogurt
- Apple slices with Fruit Dip*
- ½ cup Fun Mix,* 1 low-fat mozzarella cheese stick
- Cranberry juice (4 ounces), cream cheese on 4 whole wheat crackers
- 4 mini rice cakes topped with 1 tablespoon favorite spread

LUNCH BUNCH

- 1 Mini Chickpea Cake*
- ½ cup applesauce, ½ cup cubed cheddar cheese, 4 whole wheat crackers
- ½ cup whole wheat pasta with ½ cup peas
- 1 Honey Bran Square* cut into small bites
- 1 Peanut Spinach Ball* cut into small pieces
- 1 slice whole wheat bread with turkey breast and ranch dressing cut into small pieces
- ½ cup vanilla yogurt mixed with 1 tablespoon peanut butter, ½ cup blueberries, ¼ cup diced ham

BRAIN SNACKS

- Snack Mix* (no nuts)
- Frozen Apple Fruit Cup*
- 1 slice low-fat cheese, ½ apple, peeled and diced

- 1 graham cracker with 1 tablespoon cream cheese
- Carrot Raisin Rounds*
- ½ cup Yogurt Parfait*
- ½ cup fresh fruit cut in small pieces with 1 tablespoon ranch dressing

DINNER

- Peas and Bow Ties*
- ¼ cup spaghetti with cheese toast and ½ cup meatball cut in pieces
- ½ cup black beans and brown rice, ¼ cup applesauce
- Chicken Nuggets,* ½ cup green beans
- Tuna Burger* cut small with ranch dressing to dip
- ½ cup Cheese Spinach Noodles,* ½ cup sliced peaches
- ½ cup creamed corn and rice, 1 ounce turkey breast

chapter 4: menus for 4- to 6-year-olds

As children grow past the years of critical brain development, their nutrient needs increase proportionally to their physical growth. Therefore, more carbohydrates, protein, fat, and calories are needed in the daily diet of a child 4 to 6 years of age. In addition, your child has now entered school and is developing behavioral and learning skills—a time when wise food choices by parents for their child are important for a child's optimal mood and abilities while in the school environment. Packing a balanced lunch and snacks to send with your child to school, along with a complete breakfast before leaving the home, is the best way to ensure a happy, successful day.

The following meal plans are nutrient balanced for a child age 4 to 6. Picking one meal from each section of the day provides your child with an overall balanced diet to meet their bodies' growing needs. As you create new meal plans, be sure to balance carbohydrate food sources with protein ones. And keep the amount of fat lower than 31 percent of total daily intake. Remember that although some of the recipes or meals suggested have a higher amount of fat percentage for a single meal, it is the average of the entire day's diet that is important. For example, eating bacon and eggs in the morning (a high-fat meal) is balanced by eating a low-fat, higher-carbohydrate meal at lunchtime, such as a baked potato topped with veggies.

BREAKFAST

- Whole wheat pancakes with butter and ½ cup berries
- Breakfast Pizza*
- Scrambled eggs, 1 slice whole wheat toast, ½ cup blueberries
- Yogurt Parfait*
- On-the-Run Smoothie,* 1 slice whole wheat toast
- Sunrise Pizza*
- ½ cup oatmeal with ½ cup sliced bananas, milk

MORNING GLORIES

- Yogurt with baked chips
- Graham crackers with peanut butter and raisins
- Snack Mix*
- Fruit Smoothie*
- Pita Triangles*
- 1 Banana Roll*
- 1 cup yogurt mixed with ½ tablespoon peanut butter

LUNCH BUNCH

- Pita bread half with 1 tablespoon crunchy peanut butter and 4 apple slices
- Whole wheat bun with 1 ounce melted mozzarella cheese, a nectarine
- Sliced cucumbers with ranch dressing, bran muffin, a cheese stick
- ½ cup diced ham, ½ cup vanilla yogurt, ½ cup strawberries
- Hard-boiled egg, ½ an orange, ½ a pita with peanut butter
- Baby carrots, Applesauce Muffins,* cream cheese on 5 whole wheat crackers
- 4 ounces turkey breast slices with honey mustard in a whole wheat pita

BRAIN SNACKS

- Fresh Fruit Pizza Cookie*
- Fruit Smoothie*
- Chocolate Banana Bread*
- 1 cup of cut-up veggies, low-fat ranch dip, 8 small cubes of cheddar cheese
- Five-Fruit Salad*

- Banana Pops*
- Yogurt Parfait*

- Peanut Ginger Pasta Salad*
- Barbecue Turkey Sloppy Joes*
- Chicken Nuggets,* ¹/₂ cup cut fresh fruit, 1 tbsp. ranch dip
- ¹/₂ cup ham, ¹/₄ cup brown rice, ¹/₄ cup applesauce
- Tuna Burgers,* ¹/₂ cup cut fresh fruit, ¹/₄ cup peas
- ¹/₂ cup spaghetti, ¹/₄ cup popcorn shrimp
- Cheese Spinach Noodles,* ¹/₂ cup Spiced Banana*

CHAPTER 5: Menus for 7- to 10-year-olds

Children at this stage have developed significantly and continue to grow rapidly. They are also highly active and sleeping less than just a few years earlier. To keep up with their growth and added activity, their diet needs to provide an increased amount of calories for energy expenditure. However, not just any calories will do. Adding a second helping of dessert or doubling up on bread and rolls at lunch are not wise ways to add calories. Sure, the calorie intake will be higher, but so will the intake of sugar. Be careful to add calories that are full of nutrients and balanced between protein, fat, and carbohydrate sources.

The week of meal plans provided are high in nutrient-dense calories. A variety of food colors and food textures on a plate is a sign of a good balanced meal. Food colors are yellow, green, red, and orange. Pumpkin, carrots, apricots, and sweet potatoes are examples of yellow foods. Broccoli, kale, collard greens, and spinach are foods found in the green color group. Red food examples are strawberries, watermelon, and tomatoes. Finally, the orange color group includes grapefruit, oranges, and cantaloupe. Continue to plan meals that include a similar variety to the meal plans suggested for a continued balance in your child's diet.

BREAKFAST

- Oatmeal Pancakes*
- Breakfast Pizza*
- ¹/₂ grapefruit, 2 slices whole wheat toast with peanut butter
- Granola cereal, ¹/₂ apple sliced, 1 cup yogurt

- Egg omelet with cheese, 6 ounces orange juice
- French toast topped with fresh berries
- 4 ounces milk, Breakfast Blossoms*

MORNING GLORIES

- ¹/₂ cup blueberries, 1 slice low-fat cheese
- Peanut butter on banana slices
- Fruit Smoothie*
- Stuffed Apple Rings*
- Spicy Snakes*
- 4 ounces yogurt with ¹/₂ cup strawberries mixed in
- Cereal Trail Mix*

LUNCH BUNCH

- Pita bread half, light cream cheese, sliced cucumber, applesauce on side
- Whole wheat bun, peanut butter, apple slices
- ¹/₂ cup tuna, 1 stalk chopped celery
- 1 cup grapes, 4 whole wheat crackers with cheese, 1 cup of soup*
- 2 Ham Melts,* ¹/₂ cup mandarin orange segments
- Pizza Pita*
- Chili Blanco*

BRAIN SNACKS

- Fresh Fruit Pizza Cookie*
- Snack Mix*
- Low-fat vanilla or plain yogurt, a handful of nuts
- Cream cheese on celery
- ¹/₂ cup Waldorf salad
- Frozen Fruit Cup*
- Graham cracker with peanut butter and raisins

DINNER

- Grilled salmon, baked potato with broccoli, sour cream, and low-fat cheese
- Barbecue Turkey Sloppy Joes*
- Roasted chicken, ¹/₂ sweet potato, 1 sliced banana with cinnamon*
- Chicken Nuggets,* ¹/₂ cup five-bean salad
- Carrot Risotto,* ¹/₂ cup creamed spinach*

- 4 ounces lasagna, $\frac{1}{2}$ cup green beans, $\frac{1}{4}$ cup banana pudding
- Cheese Spinach Noodles,* $\frac{1}{2}$ cup applesauce

CHAPTER 6: menus for 11- to 14-year-olds

Children at this age are more independent now than any other time prior. They are making their own food choices as they get ready for school in the morning and while at school in the lunch line. By the time dinner is ready, they have already consumed three or four meals and snacks. The foods consumed may or may not provide preteens with the amount of energy and type of nutrients they need to perform optimally in class and on the practice field. Your control over their food choices is limited. Be sure to provide healthy snacks regularly at home. The foods in the refrigerator or freezer and on the countertop or in the cupboards need to be quick and easy to prepare.

The following meal plans can be made in a short amount of time and with few ingredients. The meals are easy enough for preteens to make for themselves. Having available quick, high-quality foods helps to ensure a more balanced daily diet. A child's diet needs to be balanced from a full day of food intake and not from one meal. Therefore, if your child eats a burger and fries for lunch while out with friends, and balances the rest of the day with higher-nutrient foods, such as an apple and yogurt, tuna salad and nuts, or a fresh fruit smoothie, your preteen is able to get the vitamins and minerals needed for optimal health.

BREAKFAST

- Oatmeal Pancakes*
- Breakfast Pizza*
- $\frac{1}{2}$ cup plain yogurt, $\frac{1}{2}$ cup blueberries, 1 slice whole wheat toast with peanut butter
- $\frac{1}{2}$ cup cheese grits, $\frac{1}{2}$ cup strawberries
- Ham Melts,* 6 ounces orange juice
- 1 slice Canadian bacon, 1 egg scrambled, 1 wheat English muffin
- On-the-Run Smoothie,* $\frac{1}{2}$ wheat bagel with cream cheese

MORNING GLORIES

- Cereal Trail Mix*
- Fruit Smoothie*
- Fun Mix*

- 2 Stuffed Apple Rings*
- 2 Banana Rolls*
- 1 apple, 1 tablespoon peanut butter
- 1 Applesauce Muffin* with $\frac{1}{2}$ cup cubed cheddar cheese on the side

LUNCH BUNCH

- Buffalo-Style Wraps*
- Club sandwich on whole wheat bread with bacon, ham, turkey, cheese, lettuce, and tomato
- Chili Blanco*
- Spinach Rice Salad*
- 2 Mini Chick Pea Cakes,* 1 cup yogurt
- Pita Pizza*
- $\frac{1}{2}$ cup fruit salad, 1 cup brown rice, 2 ounces diced turkey

BRAIN SNACKS

- Apple sliced with peanut butter as a dip
- Fruit Smoothie*
- Frozen Apple Fruit Cup*
- 1 string cheese, $\frac{1}{2}$ cup mixed nuts
- 1 Banana Roll*
- Yogurt Parfait*
- Carrot Raisin Rounds*

DINNER

- Peanut Ginger Pasta Salad*
- Barbecue Turkey Sloppy Joes,* 1 corn on the cob, $\frac{1}{2}$ cup Spiced Bananas*
- $\frac{1}{2}$ cup spaghetti, 3 ounces grilled fish, $\frac{1}{2}$ cup five-bean salad
- Tangy Citrus Chicken,* $\frac{1}{2}$ cup cut-up fresh fruit, $\frac{1}{2}$ cup coleslaw
- Sesame Shrimp and Asparagus,* $\frac{1}{2}$ cup brown rice, $\frac{1}{2}$ cup apples
- Spiced Pork Tenderloins,* $\frac{1}{2}$ cup pasta, $\frac{1}{2}$ cup Waldorf salad
- Carrot Risotto,* $\frac{1}{2}$ cup popcorn shrimp, $\frac{1}{2}$ cup side salad

chapter 7: menus for 15- to 18-year-olds

Even though the brain has completed most of its growth by adolescence, it continues to make vital connections during the teen years. This is another window of opportunity for brain growth, when a healthy diet is important. However, adolescence tends to be a time when there is a lack of essential fatty acids in the diet for many reasons. First, teens tend to eat a lot of saturated fatty foods and foods that contain hydrogenated fats. Second, due to pressure to please their peers and compete in athletics, adolescents often restrict their fat intake in order to keep fit and trim. When they cut out fat from their diets, they cut out the good with the bad fats. Teen brains need more fish and fewer fries.

The week's worth of meals listed here suggest a higher amount of fat and protein and less sugar and empty calories usually seen in a teen's diet. Take empty-calorie foods out of the kitchen and stock up on healthier options.

BREAKFAST

- Sunrise Pizza,* 1 cup milk
- Whole wheat buttermilk pancakes topped with fresh blueberries, 1 slice bacon
- Yogurt Parfait,* 2 slices whole wheat toast with 1 tablespoon peanut butter
- Slow-cooked oatmeal mixed with ½ cup sliced bananas and ½ cup sliced strawberries
- On-the-Run Smoothie*
- Cheese omelet, ½ cup cut melon fruit
- Applesauce Muffins,* ½ cup vanilla yogurt, 4 ounces orange juice

MORNING GLORIES

- 2 Honey Bran Squares*
- 1 cup yogurt with granola and berries
- 2 Applesauce Muffins*
- 1 banana with 1 tablespoon peanut butter
- Cereal Trail Mix*
- ½ cup cubed cheese with ½ cup cut strawberries
- Spicy Snakes*

LUNCH BUNCH

- Pizza Pita*
- Peachy Peanut Butter Pitas*
- Buffalo-Style Wraps*
- 1 Banana Roll,* 1 cup vanilla yogurt, 1 cup side salad with 2 ounces turkey

- Grilled Eggplant Salad*
- Sliced banana with peanut butter and raisin sandwich on whole wheat bread
- 1 cup Chili Blanco*

BRAIN SNACKS

- Carrot Raisin Rounds*
- Smoothie Pops*
- 1 cup yogurt with blueberries
- Tree Snacks*
- Stuffed Apple Rings*
- 5 whole wheat crackers with cheese
- Fruit Kabobs*

DINNER

- Peanut Ginger Pasta and Veggies*
- Barbecue Turkey Sloppy Joes*
- Tuna Burgers,* $\frac{1}{2}$ cup spaghetti, $\frac{1}{2}$ cup Waldorf salad
- 8 Chicken Nuggets,* $\frac{1}{2}$ cup fruit salad, $\frac{1}{2}$ cup brown rice
- Sesame Shrimp and Asparagus,* $\frac{1}{2}$ cup applesauce
- 4 ounces lasagna, $\frac{1}{2}$ cup green beans, $\frac{1}{2}$ cup Spiced Bananas*
- Grilled salmon, $\frac{1}{2}$ cup pasta, $\frac{1}{2}$ cup five-bean salad, side salad

Appendix C

Glossary

Aerobic: Occurring in the presence of oxygen. An aerobic activity is one in which the intensity allows adequate oxygen intake to meet tissue demands.

Amenorrhea: The absence or abnormal discontinuation of the menses.

Amino acid: An organic acid containing an amino (NH-2) group; the small building blocks of protein.

Anemia: A condition characterized by a deficiency of hemoglobin red blood cells or red blood cells that are abnormal in size, or both.

Anorexia: The lack or loss of appetite for food.

Antioxidant: A substance that prevents or impedes oxidation.

Arteriosclerosis: A variety of conditions in which the artery walls thicken and lose their elasticity. Commonly referred to as "hardening of the arteries."

Ascorbic acid: Vitamin C.

ATP: Adenosine triphosphate—the energy currency in the body.

Balanced diet: Diet supplying all known essential nutrients in optimal amounts and appropriate ratios to each other.

Basal metabolic rate (BMR): The energy required for internal or cellular work when the body is at rest.

Blood sugar: Amount of glucose in circulating blood; varies within normal limits.

Calorie: A unit of heat used in metabolic studies for energy denotation.

Carbohydrate: Heat-producing organic compounds, such as starches, cellulose, and sugars.

Cardiovascular disease: The combination of heart and blood vessel disorders that include heart attack, stroke, atherosclerosis, and congestive heart failure.

Cholesterol: A fatty substance or sterol found in all animal fats, bile, skin, blood, and brain tissues; the precursor for vitamin D and the sex hormones and important in the formation and maintenance of myelin. At elevated levels in the blood, cholesterol is a primary risk factor in cardiovascular disease.

Daily Reference Value (DRV): Set of dietary references that applies to fat, saturated fat, cholesterol, carbohydrate, fiber, protein, sodium, and potassium.

Daily Value (DV): New dietary references term made up of two sets of references, DRVs and RDIs.

Diabetes mellitus: A disorder in which the pancreas produces insufficient or no insulin or the cells are insensitive to insulin. The result is an inability to maintain normal blood sugar levels.

Disaccharide: Any sugar that yields two monosaccharides (sucrose, lactose, or maltose) when hydrolyzed.

Electrolyte: The ionized form of an ion. Common electrolytes include sodium, potassium, and chloride.

Enriched: The description of processed food that has four nutrients (thiamin, riboflavin, niacin, and iron) added back to replace partially those lost in refining.

Essential amino acid: An amino acid that cannot be synthesized by the body and must be supplied by the diet.

Essential fatty acid: A fatty acid, such as linoleic acid, that cannot be made by the body and must be supplied regularly from the diet.

Fat: Glycerol with fatty acids found in animal or vegetable origin.

Fatigue: Feelings of lethargy, tiredness, or physical and mental weariness.

Fatty acid: Open-chained monocarboxylic acid comprised of carbon, hydrogen, and oxygen.

Fiber: An indigestible complex carbohydrate found in plants; roughage.

Food allergen: Substances in food, or foods themselves, that could cause disorders or negative reactions in the body when ingested.

Food guide pyramid: Guidelines of recommended amounts and types of foods a diet should include.

Fortification: The addition of one or more nutrients to a food in greater amounts than naturally found.

Fructose: A monosaccharide composed of six-carbon sugar; found in fruits and honey and obtained by hydrolysis of sucrose or table sugar; also called fruit sugar.

Galactose: A monosaccharide resulting from the hydrolysis of lactose.

Glucose: The monosaccharide found in fruits and sugars that forms starch when linked in long strands; the storage of body sugar; the sugar found in blood.

HDL cholesterol: Type of cholesterol packaged in high-density lipoproteins. High levels of HDL are associated with a lower risk of cardiovascular disease.

Homeostasis: The body's regulatory mechanism that tries to maintain stability and consistency in the various systems, such as body temperature, fluid volume, and concentration of electrolytes.

Hormone: A specific chemical substance secreted by an endocrine gland through the blood to regulate functions of tissues and organs elsewhere in the body.

Insulin: A hormone produced by the pancreas that regulates blood sugar levels.

Korsakoff's disease: A syndrome characterized by confusion, amnesia, and apathy; seen in alcoholics and other B vitamin–deficient individuals.

Kwashiorkor: A protein deficiency disease seen in malnourished children and characterized by growth failure, edema, tissue wasting, decreased resistance to illness, and pigment changes in the skin.

Lactose: A disaccharide found in milk and composed of galactose and glucose.

LDL cholesterol: Low-density lipoprotein. A compound comprised of fat and protein that transports fats in the blood. High levels of this type of cholesterol are associated with an increased risk of cardiovascular disease.

Legume: The seed or fruit of a pod-bearing plant, including dried peas, and beans, lentils, and chickpeas.

Lipid: A term for the family of fats including triglycerides, cholesterol, and phospholipids.

Macronutrients: The nutrients that the body requires in relatively large amounts, including protein, carbohydrate, fats, and water.

Maltose: A disaccharide composed of two glucose units.

Menstruation: The monthly discharge of blood and tissue from the uterus occurring between puberty and menopause.

Metabolism: The sum total of all anabolic and catabolic chemical reactions within the body.

Micronutrients: The nutrients required by the body in relatively small amounts, including vitamins and minerals.

Mineral: Inorganic materials, like iron or copper, necessary in small amounts for the functioning of the body and brain.

MSG: Monosodium glutamine; a food additive that produces adverse reactions in sensitive individuals.

Neuron: A nerve cell that transmits electrical impulses, causing the release of neurotransmitters.

Neurotransmitter: A chemical that serves as a communication link between neurons.

Nonessential amino acids: Amino acids that are necessary for growth and maintenance but that can be synthesized by the body from amino acids and other molecules.

Nutrient: A substance serving as or providing nourishment.

Nutrient density: The ratio of nutrients to calories supplied by a food. Foods that provide a substantial amount of nutrients and few calories are considered nutrient dense.

Obesity: Body fat 20 percent or more above the ideal.

Polysaccharide: Complex carbohydrates or starches; formed from strings of glucose units.

PMS: Premenstrual syndrome; a group of physical and emotional symptoms affecting women the week or two prior to menstruation.

Protein: Built up of amino acids; necessary for growth and repair of the body.

Reference Daily Intake (RDI): Set of dietary references based on RDAs for essential vitamins and minerals (and protein in select groups). "RDI" replaces "U.S. RDA."

Recommended Dietary Allowance (RDA): Set of estimated allowances established by the National Academy of Sciences. Updated periodically to reflect current scientific knowledge.

Salt sensitive: Describes individuals who experience a change in blood pressure in response to a high or low salt intake.

Satiety: A feeling of satisfaction following eating.

Saturated fat: A fat or fatty acid containing the maximum number of hydrogen atoms.

Serotonin: A neurotransmitter formed from the amino acid tryptophan that regulates mood, sleep, appetite, and pain.

Steroid: A group of compounds structurally similar to cholesterol, including bile acids, sterols, and sex hormones.

Synapse: The junction between two neurons where a nervous impulse is transmitted from one neuron to the next.

Thiamin: Vitamin B1.

Triglycerides: Fatty compounds composed of one glycerol and three fatty acid molecules.

Unsaturated fat: A fat that has one or more double bonds and could accept additional hydrogens.

Vitamin: Biochemicals vital in small quantities for the vital processes in the body and brain.

Appendix D

nutritional tables and charts

TABLE 1. The carbohydrate content of common American foods, including grams and percentages for specific servings

Food Type	Sample Portion	Grams per Serving	Grams of Carbo-hydrate Percent	Carbo-hydrate by Weight
Complex Carbohydrates				
Bread, all kinds	1 slice	25	13	50–56
Cereals, breakfast, dry	1 cup wheat flakes	30	24	68–84
Crackers, all kinds	4 saltines	11	8	67–73
Flour, all kinds	2 tablespoons	14	11	71–80
Legumes, dry	½ cup navy beans, cooked	95	20	60–63
Macaroni, spaghetti, dry	½ cup cooked	70	16	75
Nuts	¼ cup peanuts	36	7	15–20
Pie crust, baked	⅙ shell	30	13	44
Potatoes, white, raw	1 boiled	122	18	17
Rice, dry	½ cup cooked	105	25	80

(continued)

TABLE 1. The carbohydrate content of common American foods, including grams and percentages for specific servings (continued)

Food Type	Sample Portion	Grams per Serving	Grams of Carbo- hydrate Percent	Carbo- hydrate by Weight
Complex and Simple Carbohydrates				
Cake, plain and iced	1 piece layer, iced	75	45	52–68
Cookies	1 chocolate chip	10	6	51–80
Simple Carbohydrates				
Beverages, carbonated	8 ounces cola	246	24	8–12
Candy (without nuts)	1 ounce milk chocolate	28	16	75–95
Fruit, dried	4 prunes	32	18	59–60
Fruit, fresh	1 apple	150	18	6–22
Fruit, sweetened, canned or frozen	½ cup peaches	128	26	16–28
Ice cream	½ cup	67	14	18–21
Milk	1 cup	244	12	5
Pudding	½ cup vanilla	128	21	16–26
Sugar, all kinds	1 tablespoon white	11	11	96–100
Syrups, molasses, honey	1 tablespoon molasses	20	13	65–82
Vegetables	½ cup green beans	63	4	4–18

TABLE 2. Protein requirements

Group	RDA (g)
Infants (age in months)	
0–6 (13 lbs.)	13
6–12 (20 lbs.)	14
Children (age in years)	
1–3 (29 lbs.)	16
4–6 (44 lbs.)	24
7–10 (62 lbs.)	28
11–14 (99 lbs.)	45
15–18 (145 lbs.)	59

TABLE 3. High-fiber foods

Food Source	Fiber (g)
Apple	3.6
Dried figs	3.5
Carrots	3.1
Broccoli	2.9
Spinach	2.8
Orange	2.6
Prunes	2.0
Blueberries	2.0
Peach	1.9

Source: *Journal of the American Dietetic Association* 86 (1986): 732.

TABLE 4. Protein content of foods, based on averages for food types

Food	Average Serving	Protein (g)
Milk Group		
Milk, whole or skim	1 c.	9
Nonfat dry milk	7/8 oz. (3–5 tbsp.)	9
Cottage cheese	2 oz.	10
American cheese	1 oz.	7
Ice cream	1/8 qt.	3
Meat Group		
Meat, fish, poultry	3 oz., cooked	15–25
Egg	1 whole	6
Dried beans or peas	1/2 c. cooked	7–8
Peanut butter	1 tbsp.	4
Vegetable-Fruit Group		
Vegetables	1/2 c.	1–3
Fruits	1/2 c.	12
Bread and Cereals Group		
Breakfast cereals, wheat	1/2 c. cooked	2–3
	1/4 c. dry	2–3
Bread, wheat	1 slice	2–3
Macaroni, noodles, spaghetti	1/2 c. cooked	2
Rice	1/2 c. cooked	2
Cornmeal and cereal	1/2 c. cooked	2

BRAIN FOOD

TABLE 5. Percentage of fat calories in selected foods

Food	Amount	Fat Calories	Total Calories	Percent Fat
Beverages				
Beer, wine	1 serving	0	85–150	0
Coffee, tea	1 serving	0	0	0
Fruit, juice	6 oz.	0	75–110	0
Dairy Products				
Milk, chocolate cocoa mix	1 c.	108	245	44
Milk, whole	1 c.	81	160	50
2 percent	1 c.	45	145	31
Nonfat	1 c.	Trace	90	<1
Buttermilk	1 c.	Trace	90	<1
Cheese				
Cheddar	1 oz.	1	115	70
Cottage, creamed	1 c.	90	260	35
Cottage, uncreamed	1 c.	9	170	5.3
Cream	1 cu. in.	54	60	90
Parmesan	1 oz.	81	130	2
Swiss	1 oz.	72	104	69
Processed	1 oz.	81	105	77
Cheese food	1 tbsp.	27	45	60
Cream,				
half & half	1 c.	252	325	78
sour	1 c.	423	485	87
Whipping, light	1 c.	675	715	95
Whipping, heavy	1 c.	810	840	96
Imitation creamers				
Powdered	1 tsp.	9	10	90
Liquid	1 tbsp.	18	20	90
Custard	1 c.	135	305	44
Ice cream	1 c.	126	255	49
Ice milk	1 c.	63	200	31
Yogurt, low fat	1 c.	36	125	29
Whole	1 c.	72	150	49

(continued)

Food	Amount	Fat Calories	Total Calories	Percent Fat
Meat, Poultry, Fish/Shellfish; Related Products				
Bacon	2 slices	72	90	80
Beef				
Hamburger				
Regular	3 oz.	153	245	63
Lean	3 oz.	90	185	49
Steak, broiled				
(lean only)	2 oz.	36	115	31
(lean and fat)	3 oz.	243	330	74
Roast, oven-cooked				
Rib (lean only)	1.8 oz.	63	125	50
(lean and fat)	3 oz.	306	375	81
Roast, oven-cooked				
heel of round				
(lean only)	2.7 oz.	27	125	22
(lean and fat)	3 oz.	63	165	38
Canned, corned	3 oz.	90	185	49
Chicken, flesh only				
(broiled)	3 oz.	27	115	23
Drumstick (fried)	2.1	36	90	40
Chili con carne				
with beans	1 c.	135	335	40
without beans	1 c.	342	510	67
Pork				
Ham, light cured	3 oz.	171	245	70
Luncheon, ham	2 oz.	90	135	67
Roast pork	3 oz.	216	310	70
Sausage	1 oz.	63	90	70
Bologna	2 slices	63	80	79
Fish				
Clams	3 oz.	9	45	20
Crab meat	3 oz.	18	85	21
Oysters	1 c.	36	160	23
Salmon	3 oz.	45	120	38

TABLE 5. Percentage of fat calories in selected foods (continued)

Food	Amount	Fat Calories	Total Calories	Percent Fat
Shrimp	3 oz.	9	100	9
Tuna				
Canned in oil	3 oz.	63	170	37
Mature Beans, Peas, Nuts; Related Products				
Almonds	1 c.	693	850	82
Beans				
Great Northern	1 c.	9	210	4
Navy	1 c.	9	225	4
Cashews	1 c.	576	785	73
Peanuts	1 c.	648	840	77
Peas, split	1 c.	9	290	3
Vegetables				
Asparagus through zucchini		Trace		<1
Exceptions:				
Candied sweet potatoes	1	63	295	21
All fried, sautéed, or buttered vegetables				
Fruits				
Apples through watermelon		Trace		<1
Exception:				
Avocado	1	333	370	90
Grain Products				
Breads and cereals				<12
Exceptions:				
Biscuits	1	45	105	43
Cupcake	1	27	90	30
Devil's food cake	1 piece	81	235	35

(continued)

TABLE 5. Percentage of fat calories in selected foods (continued)

Food	Amount	Fat Calories	Total Calories	Percent Fat
Gingerbread	⅛ of 8"	36	175	20
Fruitcake	1 slice	18	55	33
Cookies	1	27	50	54
Brownies	1	54	95	57
Corn muffins	1	36	125	29
Crackers (saltines)	4	9	50	18
Danish pastry	1	135	275	49
Pancakes	1	18	60	30
Waffles	1	63	210	30
All fats: butter, lard, vegetable oils, shortening, margarine, salad dressing, mayonnaise, and chicken fat				100

TABLE 6. Cholesterol content of foods

Food	Amount	Cholesterol (mg)
Liver	3 oz.	372
Egg	1	252
Ladyfingers	4	157
Custard	½ c.	139
Sardines	3¼ oz.	129
Apple or custard pie	⅛ of 9" pie	120
Waffles, mix, egg, milk	1 (9" × 9")	112
Lemon meringue pie	⅛ of 9" pie	98
Veal	3 oz.	86
Turkey, dark meat, no skin	3 oz.	86
Lamb	3 oz.	83
Beef	3 oz.	80
Pork	3 oz.	76
Spaghetti, meatballs	1 c.	75

Table 6. Cholesterol content of foods (continued)

Food	Amount	Cholesterol (mg)
Lobster	3 oz.	72
Turkey, light meat, no skin	3 oz.	65
Chicken breast	½ breast	63
Noodles, whole egg	1 c., cooked	50
Clams	½ c.	50
Macaroni and cheese	1 c.	42
Chicken drumstick	1	39
Oysters	3 oz.	38
Fish fillet	3 oz.	34–75
Whole milk	8 oz.	34
Salmon, canned	3 oz.	30
Hot dog	1	27
Cheddar or Swiss cheese	1 oz.	28
Rice pudding with raisins	1 c.	29
Ice cream	½ c.	27–49
American processed cheese	1 oz.	25
Low-fat milk (2%)	8 oz.	22
Heavy whipping cream	1 tbsp.	20
Mozzarella, part skim	1 oz.	18
Brownies ($1^3/_4$" × $1^3/_4$" × $1^1/_8$")	1	17
Yogurt, plain	8 oz.	17
Cream cheese	1 tbsp.	16
Cottage cheese	½ c.	12–24
Butter	1 pat/tsp.	12
Mayonnaise	1 tbsp.	10
Sour cream	1 tbsp.	8
Half-and-half	1 tbsp.	6
Cottage cheese, dry curd	½ c.	6
Non-fat milk/buttermilk	8 oz.	5
Margarine		0
Beans, grains, nuts, fruits, vegetables		0

TABLE 7. Vitamin and mineral safety issues

Nutrient	RDI	Toxic Dose	Symptoms
Vitamin A	5,000 IU	50,000–500,000 UI	Chronic ingestion of the less amount can cause headache and nausea, while a single extremely high dose can cause acute, reversible effects.
Beta-carotene	10–30 mg[a]	——	High intakes are not associated with any toxicity symptoms. Hypercarotenemia (harmless yellowing of the skin) might occur with large intakes.
Vitamin D	400 IU	25,000–200,000 IU	Nausea, vomiting, loss of appetite, dry mouth, headache, and dizziness can occur.
Vitamin E	30 IU	3,000 IU	Safe, even with prolonged, high intakes. Individuals on anticoagulants should avoid doses above 400 UI.
Vitamin B1	1.5 mg	——	Excesses cleared by kidneys, generally considered safe at all intake levels.
Vitamin B2	1.7 mg	——	No reported toxic effects.
Niacin	20 mg	300–600 mg	Headache, nausea, and skin (niacinamide form) blotching can occur. Flushing, rashes, tingling (nicotinic acid form) and itching can occur. Doses exceeding 2.5 grams/day can cause liver damage and glucose intolerance.
Vitamin B6	2 mg	250–1,000 mg	Prolonged high doses can cause reversible nerve damage.
Vitamin B12	4 mcg	——	No reported toxic effects.
Folacin	400 mcg	400–1,000 mcg	Safe up to 15 mg. However, lower doses can increase excretion of zinc and mask symptoms of vitamin B12 deficiency.

TABLE 7. Vitamin and mineral safety issues (continued)

Nutrient	RDI	Toxic Dose	Symptoms
Pantothenic acid	10 mg	10–20 mg	Generally safe at high doses; can produce diarrhea and water retention.
Vitamin C	60 mg	1,000–5,000 mg	Some research shows no toxicity at intakes as high as 10,000 mg/day. Doses as low as 1,000–2,000 mg might contribute to kidney stones, mineral interactions, impaired immune function, and withdrawal symptoms.
Calcium	1,000 mg	3,000–8,000 mg	Numerous adverse symptoms, including nausea, vomiting, high blood pressure, diarrhea, constipation, and milk-alkali syndrome.
Chromium	50–200 mcg[b]	——	No known or reported toxic effects.
Copper	2 mg	——	Nausea, vomiting, headache, jaundice.
Iron	18 mg	18+ mg	Constipation and stomach upset can occur. Doses above 100 mg daily can result in abdominal pain, fatigue, weight loss, and possibly heart disease.
Magnesium	400 mg	1,000+ mg	Diarrhea, low blood pressure, and nausea can occur.
Selenium	50–200 mcg[b]	800–3,000 mcg	Brittle hair and fingernails, dizziness, fatigue, nausea, diarrhea, and liver disease can occur.
Zinc	15 mg	5–15 mg	Can interfere with copper absorption, lower HDL-cholesterol, impair immune response, and cause dizziness, vomiting, and anemia.

[a] There is no established RDA for beta-carotene. This intake is recommended by the Alliance for Aging Research.
[b] Estimated Safe and Adequate Daily Dietary Intake.

TABLE 8. Supplement label terms

Chelated minerals: A chelated mineral is chemically bound to another substance, usually an amino acid; such as iron/amino chelate or chromium proteinate. Chelation is claimed to improve mineral absorption, but there is little proof of this advantage. However, chelated minerals might be less irritating to the stomach and intestine.

Time released: Time-released supplements were developed to dissolve slowly in the intestine, increase the amount of absorption of a vitamin or mineral, and hopefully reduce dramatic fluctuations in blood levels. However, most time-released tablets dissolve too slowly to be completely absorbed. The time-release forms of niacin are well absorbed but might increase the risk of liver damage. Therapeutic doses of niacin should be monitored by a physician (M.D.).

Natural versus synthetic: Supplements labeled "natural" or "organic" are often no different from other supplements—except in price. The body cannot distinguish between a natural and synthetic nutrient and many "natural" products are actually synthetic vitamins mixed with small amounts of "natural" vitamins.

The exceptions are selenium, chromium, and vitamin E. "Organic" selenium, called selenium-rich yeast or L-selenomethionine, and chromium, called chromium-rich yeast, are better absorbed and used by the body than their inorganic forms, such as sodium selenite and chromic chloride. Body tissues prefer the "natural" form of vitamin E, called d-alpha tocopherol, to the synthetic counterpart, called dl-alpha tocopherol or all-rac alpha tocopherol.

Buffered: The acidity of some vitamins, such as vitamin C, can irritate the digestive tract when consumed in large doses. A compound that buffers or neutralizes the acidity of a nutrient can be added to a supplement and counteract the irritating effects. For example, ascorbate is the buffered form of vitamin C.

Table 9. Fiber content of major food groups identified by soluble and insoluble components

	Serving size (*½ c. cooked) (unless otherwise indicated)	Total fiber (g)	Soluble fiber (g)	Insoluble fiber (g)
Breads, Cereals				
Bran (100%) cereal	*	10.0	0.3	9.7
Popcorn	3 c.	2.8	0.8	2.0
Rye bread	1 slice	2.7	0.8	1.9
Whole grain bread	1 slice	2.7	0.08	2.8
Rye wafers	3	2.3	0.06	2.2
Corn grits	*	1.9	0.6	1.3
Oats, whole	*	1.6	0.5	1.1
Graham crackers	2	1.4	0.04	1.4
Brown rice	*	1.3	0	1.3
French bread	1 slice	1.0	0.4	0.6
Dinner roll	1	0.8	0.03	0.8
Egg noodles	*	0.8	0.3	0.8
Spaghetti	*	0.8	0.02	0.8
White bread	1 slice	0.8	0.03	0.8
White rice	*	0.5	0	0.5

	Serving size (raw)	Total fiber (g)	Soluble fiber (g)	Insoluble fiber (g)
Fruits				
Apples	1 small	3.9	2.3	1.6
Blackberries	½ c.	3.7	0.7	3.0
Pear	1 small	2.5	0.6	1.9
Strawberries	¾ c.	2.4	0.9	1.5
Plums	2 medium	2.3	1.3	1.0
Tangerine	1 medium	1.6	1.4	0.4
Apricots	2 medium	1.3	0.9	0.4
Banana	1 small	1.3	0.6	0.7
Grapefruit	½	1.3	0.9	0.4

(continued)

	Serving size (raw)	Total fiber (g)	Soluble fiber (g)	Insoluble fiber (g)
Peaches	1 med	1.0	0.5	0.5
Cherries	10	0.9	0.3	0.6
Pineapple	½ cup	0.8	0.2	0.6
Grapes	10	0.4	0.1	0.3

	Serving size (*½ c. cooked) (unless otherwise indicated)	Total fiber (g)	Soluble fiber (g)	Insoluble fiber (g)
Legumes				
Kidney beans	*	4.5	0.5	4.0
White beans	*	4.2	0.4	3.8
Pinto beans	*	3.0	0.3	2.7
Lima beans	*	1.4	0.2	1.2
Nuts				
Almonds	10	1.0		
Peanuts	10	1.0		
Walnuts, black	1 tsp. chopped	0.6		
Pecans	2	0.5		
Vegetables				
Peas	*	5.2	2.0	3.2
Parsnips	*	4.4	.04	4.0
Potatoes	1 small	3.8	2.2	1.6
Broccoli	*	2.6	1.6	1.0
Zucchini	*	2.5	1.1	1.4
Squash, summer	*	2.3	1.1	1.2
Lettuce	½ c. raw	0.5	0.2	0.3

TABLE 10. Dietary fiber in foods

Food	Amount	Dietary Fiber (g)
Milk and Milk Products		0
Vegetables		
Asparagus	4 medium spears	0.9
Avocado	1/2 whole	2.2
Beets, boiled	1/2 c.	2.1
Broccoli	1/2 c.	3.2
Brussels sprouts	1/2 c.	2.3
Cabbage, boiled	1/2 c.	2.0
Carrots, boiled	1/2 c.	2.3
Raw	1	2.3
Celery, raw	1 stalk	0.7
Corn, off the cob	1/3 c.	3.1
On the cob	1 ear	5.9
Eggplant, peeled, cooked	1/2 c.	2.5
Lettuce	1/6 head	1.4
	6 medium leaves	0.7
Mushrooms, raw	1/2 c.	0.9
Peas, boiled	1/2 c.	4.2
Potato, baked with skin	1 medium	3.0
Boiled, peeled	1 medium	2.7
French fried	10	1.6
Mashed with milk	1/2 c.	0.9
Spinach, cooked	1/2 c.	5.7
Sweet potato, cooked	1 5" × 2"	3.5
Tomato, raw	1 medium	2.0
Juice		0
Sauce	1/2 c.	2.6
Fruits		
Apple, with peel	1 medium	3.3
Juice		0
Sauce	1/2 c.	2.6
Apricots	2 medium	1.6
Banana	1/2 medium	1.6

(continued)

TABLE 10. Dietary fiber in foods (continued)

Food	Amount	Dietary Fiber (g)
Cantaloupe	1/4	1.6
Dates, dried	5	3.1
Fig, dried	1 medium	2.4
Grapefruit, fresh	1/2 whole	0.6
Grapes, seedless	12	0.3
Nectarine	1 medium	3.0
Orange	1 small	2.4
Peach, fresh	1 medium	1.4
Pear, fresh	1 medium	2.6
Pineapple, fresh	1/2 c.	0.9
Prunes, uncooked	2 medium	2.0
Raisins	2 tbsp.	1.2
Raspberries	1/2 c.	4.6
Strawberries	1/2 c.	1.7

Bread and Cereals

Bread

Cracked wheat	1 slice	2.1
Frankfurter bun	1	1.2
Hamburger bun	1	1.2
Pumpernickel	1 slice	1.2
Raisin	1 slice	0.4
Rye	1 slice	1.2
White	1 slice	0.8
Whole wheat	1 slice	2.1

Cereals

All-Bran	1/3 c.	9.0
Bran Buds	1/3 c.	8.0
Cracklin' Bran	1/3 c.	4.0
Raisin Bran	1/3 c.	4.0

Crackers

Rye	3 3 1/2"	2.3
Saltines	4 squares	0

TABLE 10. Dietary fiber in foods (continued)

Food	Amount	Dietary Fiber (g)
Miscellaneous		
Popcorn	1 c.	0.4
Beans, baked	1/2 c.	11.0
Chili with beans	1/2 c.	8.6
Meats		0
Eggs		0
Fats (dressings, margarine, mayonnaise, etc.)		0
Nuts		
Peanut butter	2 tbsp.	2.4
Peanuts, roasted	1/4 c.	2.9
Spanish peanuts	10	0.7
Walnuts, chopped	1/4 c.	1.6

TABLE 11. Daily Recommended Values (DRVs)

Nutrient	DRV
Total fat	65 g
Saturated fat	20 g
Cholesterol	300 mg
Total carbohydrates	300 g
Dietary fiber	25 g
Sodium	2,400 mg
Potassium	3,500 mg
Protein	50 g

(continued)

TABLE 11. Daily Recommended Values (DRVs) (continued)

Nutrient	RDI (Adults and Children 4 or more years of age)	Infants	Children under 4	Pregnant and/or Lactating Women
Vitamin A	**5,000 IU**	1,500 IU	2,500 IU	8,000 IU
Vitamin C	**60 mg**	35 mg	40 mg	60 mg
Vitamin D	**400 IU**	400 IU	400 IU	400 IU
Vitamin E	**30 IU**	5 IU	10 IU	30 IU
Vitamin K	**80 mcg**	*	*	*
Thiamin (vitamin B1)	**1.5 mg**	0.5 mg	0.7 mg	1.7 mg
Riboflavin (vitamin B2)	**1.7 mg**	0.6 mg	0.8 mg	2.0 mg
Niacin	**20 mg**	8 mg	9 mg	20 mg
Vitamin B6	**2.0 mg**	0.4 mg	0.7 mg	2.5 mg
Folate (folacin, folic acid)	**400 mcg**	100 mcg	200 mcg	800 mcg
Vitamin B12	**6 mcg**	2 mcg	3 mcg	8 mcg
Biotin	**300 mcg**	50 mcg	150 mcg	300 mcg
Pantothenic acid	**10 mg**	3 mg	5 mg	10 mg
Calcium	**1,000 mg**	600 mg	800 mg	1300 mg
Iron	**18 mg**	15 mg	10 mg	18 mg
Phosphorus	**1,000 mg**	500 mg	800 mg	1300 mg
Iodine	**150 mcg**	45 mcg	70 mcg	150 mcg
Magnesium	**400 mg**	70 mg	200 mcg	450 mcg
Zinc	**15 mg**	5 mg	8 mg	15 mg
Selenium	**70 mg**	*	*	*
Copper	**2.0 mg**	0.6 mg	1.0 mg	2.0 mg
Manganese	**2.0 mg**	*	*	*
Chromium	**120 mcg**	*	*	*
Molybdenum	**75 mcg**	*	*	*
Chloride	**3,400 mg**	*	*	*
Sodium	**2,400 mg**	*	*	*
Potassium	**3,500 mg**	*	*	*

Note: **Bold type** indicates DVs based on 2,000-calorie diet for adults and children 4 or more years of age. An asterisk (*) indicates that a daily value has not been established.

TABLE 12. Summary of fat-soluble vitamins

Vitamin	Best Food Source	RDA (1989)[a]	ODA[b]	Principal Functions	Major Deficiency Symptoms
A (retinol; retinal = aldehyde form; precursors = carotenes)	Whole milk, vitamin A–fortified skim milk, butter, yellow and dark green vegetables, and orange fruits	1,000 mcg RD	10,000–35,000 IU	Maintenance of epithelial tissues; constituent of visual pigments; antioxidant	Nyctalopia, xerophthalmia, hyperkeratosis; faulty tooth formation
Carotenoids (the carotenes, the xanthophylls, and lycopene)	Orange or dark green vegetables and orange fruits	—	10–30 mg	Antioxidant; enhances cell communication and immuno-competence	Possible increased risk of cancer; impaired immunity
D (cholecalciferol = D3; ergocalci-ferol = D2)	Fish liver oils; fortified or irradiated milk	10 mcg	200–400 IU	Transport of calcium; intestinal and renal absorption and phosphate	Rickets (children); osteomalacia and possibly osteoporosis (adults)

(continued)

TABLE 12. Summary of fat-soluble vitamins (continued)

Vitamin	Best Food Source	RDA (1989)[a]	ODA[b]	Principal Functions	Major Deficiency Symptoms
E (d-alpha tocopherol)	Vegetable oils; wheat germ; dark green leafy vegetables	10 mg (alpha TE)	50–400 IU	Protects cell membranes against lipid peroxidation and destruction	Hemolytic anemia; degenerative changes in muscle; possible increased risk for heart disease and cancer
K (phylloquinone = K1; menaquinones = K2)	Green leafy vegetables, liver	70 mcg	—	Required for proper blood clotting	Hemorrhagic disease in newborn and in biliary disease; anemia

[a]Recommended Dietary Allowance for American men, 19 to 22 years of age, of average activity.

[b]Optimal Daily Allowance is a theoretical range based on the authors' literature research. If no range is listed, the authors felt that there was insufficient evidence to make a recommendation at this time.

TABLE 13. Summary of water-soluble vitamins

Vitamin	Best Food Source	RDA (1989)[a]	ODA[b]	Principal Functions	Major Deficiency Symptoms
B₁ (thiamin)	Pork, liver, yeast, whole or enriched grains, legumes	1.5 mg	5–10 mg	Decarboxylation and transketolation	Beriberi (polyneuritis), cardiovascular problems; anorexia, nausea; fatigue, paralysis
B₂ (riboflavin)	Milk, organ meats, animal protein, enriched grains, brewer's yeast	1.7 mg	6–15 mg	Coenzyme of electron transfer systems; cell respiration; metabolism of carbo-hydrates, fat, protein	Cracks and sores at corner of mouth (cheilosis), dermatitis, conjunctivitis, photophobia, glossitis
Niacin (nicotinic acid, niacinamide)	Meat, enriched or whole grains, poultry, fish, peanuts, milk products	19 mg equivalent (1 mg equivalent per 60 mg Tryp)	25–100 mg	Coenzyme of electron transfer; dehydro-genase reactions; oxidation to produce ATP (NDA+); biosyn-thesis of fatty acids, steroids, etc. (NADP+)	Pellagra, diarrhea, scaly dermatitis, dementia, stomatitis

(continued)

TABLE 13. Summary of water-soluble vitamins (continued)

Vitamin	Best Food Source	RDA (1989)[a]	ODA[b]	Principal Functions	Major Deficiency Symptoms
B6 (pyridoxine)	Meat, whole grains, poultry, fish	2.0 mg	10–20 mg	Coenzyme in amino acids metabolism; transamination, decarboxylation, transsulfuration, tryptophan synthetase, amino acid transport	Cheilosis, glossitis, stomatitis, seborrheic dermatitis, convulsions, anemia
Folacin (folic acid, peteroylglutamic acid)	Liver, greens, mushrooms, whole grains, legumes	200 mcg	400 mcg	Transfer of 1-carbon fragments (formyl); biosynthesis of purines, choline, methionine, etc.	Macrocytic and megaloblastic anemias, sprue, malabsorption, leucopenia, thrombocytopenia, birth defects
B12 (cobalamin)	Animal protein, meats, milk, egg	2 mcg	10–100 mcg	Transfer of 1-carbon fragments (methyl); biosynthesis or purines, choline, methionine, etc.; mutase reactions.	Pernicious anemia, neurological lesions, sprue

	Source	RDA[a]	Optimal Daily Allowance[b]	Function	Deficiency symptoms
Biotin	Egg yolk, organ meats, yeast, whole grains, nuts; widely distributed	30–300 mcg[c]		Acylation reactions (acetyl group transfers)	Dermatitis, alopecia, anemia; experimentally only in humans
Pantothenic acid	Liver, meat, cereal, milk, legumes; widely distributed	4.7 mg[c]	10–50 mg	Acylation reactions (acetyl group transfers)	Anemia, achromotrichia; human deficiency most unlikely
C (l-ascorbic acid)	Citrus fruits, tomatoes	60 mg	250–1,000 mg	Collagen formation; capillary walls; metabolism of Tyr, Phe, folacin, antioxidant; iron absorption	Scurvy, petechial, hemorrhages, anemia, delayed wound healing, bone fragility

[a]Recommended Dietary Allowance for American men, 19 to 22 years of age, of average activity.

[b]Optimal Daily Allowance is a theoretical range based on the authors' literature research. If no range is listed, the authors felt that there was insufficient evidence to make a recommendation at this time.

[c]Estimated safe and adequate range.

TABLE 14. Summary of the macrominerals: Calcium, magnesium, phosphorus, and the electrolytes

Mineral	Best Food Source	RDA (1989)[a]	ODA[b]	Principal Functions	Major Deficiency Symptoms
Calcium	Milk, milk products, bonemeal, dark green leafy vegetables	1,200 mg	1,000–1,500 mg	Formation of bones, teeth; blood clotting; cell membrane permeability; prevention of hypertension; neuromuscular activity	Poor growth; osteoporosis; muscle cramps
Chloride	Animal foods, table salt	750 mg[b]	—	Electrolyte balance; gastric acid; acid–base balance	Hypochloric alkalosis
Magnesium	Nuts, legumes, whole grains	350 mg (male); 280 mg (female)	400–600 mg	Constituent of bones, teeth; decreases neuromuscular sensitivity; enzyme cofactor; prevention of heart arrhythmias	Muscular tremor; confusion; vasodilation; hypertension and arrhythmias

Mineral	Sources			Functions	Deficiency/Toxicity
Phosphorus	Milk, milk products, egg yolk, meat, grains, legumes, nuts, soda pop	1,200 mg	800–1,200 mg	Formation of bones, teeth; constituent of neucleoproteins, phospholipids, phosphoproteins,	Osteomalacia. renal rickets; cardiac arrhythmias
Potassium	Vegetables, fruits, whole grains, milk legumes	2,000 mg[b]	—	Acid–base balance, water balance, CO_2 transport, cell membrane permeability, neuromuscular activity	Acidosis; renal damage; cardiac arrest

(continued)

TABLE 14. Summary of the macrominerals: Calcium, magnesium, phosphorus, and the electrolytes (continued)

Mineral	Best Food Source	RDA (1989)[a]	ODA[b]	Principal Functions	Major Deficiency Symptoms
Sodium	Table salt, salty foods, baking soda, convenience foods	500 mg[b]	—	Acid-base balance, water balance, CO_2 transport, cell membrane permeability, muscle activity	Dehydration, acidosis

[a]Recommended Dietary Allowances are established by the Food and Nutrition Board of the National Research Council. The values given are for a normal adult male, 19 to 22 years old.

[b]An estimated range recommended by the Food and Nutrition Board (1989) as safe and adequate daily intakes for healthy people.

[c]Optimal Daily Intake is a theoretical range based on the authors' literature research. If no range is listed, the authors felt there was insufficient evidence to make a recommendation at this time.

Table 15. Best sources of calcium

Best Dairy Sources	Milligrams
Yogurt, nonfat, plain (1 c.)	450
Yogurt, low-fat, plain (1 c.)	400
Yogurt, nonfat, fruit (1 c.)	300
Parmesan cheese (1 oz.)	336
Milk, low-fat (1 c.)	300
Romano cheese (1 oz.)	302
Cheddar cheese (1 oz.)	200
Cottage cheese (1 c.)	155
Sardines (3 oz.)	371
Orange juice, calcium-fortified (1 c.)	300
Rhubarb ($^1/_2$ c.)	174
Tofu (3 oz.)	190
Salmon (3 oz., canned)	180
Blackstrap molasses (1 tbsp.)	172
Figs (5)	135
Amaranth flour ($^1/_2$ c.)	150
Artichoke (1 medium)	135
Beans ($^1/_2$ c., baked)	75
Broccoli ($^1/_2$ c., chopped)	47
Collards ($^1/_2$ c., chopped)	180
Soybean nuts ($^1/_4$ c.)	116
Kale ($^1/_2$ c., chopped)	90
Okra ($^1/_2$ c.)	77
Tempeh ($^1/_2$ c.)	77
Spinach ($^1/_2$ c., canned)	136
Turnip greens ($^1/_2$ c., chopped)	100
Beet greens ($^1/_2$ c., boiled)	82
Almonds (1 oz.)	80
Almond butter (2 tbsp.)	86
Cereal, calcium fortified ($^1/_2$ c.)	100–200
Bok choy (Chinese cabbage) ($^1/_2$ c.)	79
Orange (1 medium)	50
Papaya (1 medium)	73
Sesame seeds (1 oz.)	280

TABLE 16. Essential trace minerals

Mineral	Best Food Source	RDA (1989)[a]	ODA[b]	Principal Functions	Major Deficiency Symptoms
Chromium	Whole grain breads and cereals, brewer's yeast, wheat germ, orange juice	50–200 mcg	200 mcg	Necessary for glucose utilization; possible cofactor for insulin	Unknown; deficiency linked to diabetes, decreased glucose tolerance, and cardio-vascular disease
Cobalt	Vitamin B12-rich meats, chicken, fish, milk products	—	—	Constituent of vitamin B12	Anemia
Copper	Organ meats, egg yolk, whole grain breads and cereals, legumes	1.5–3.0 mg[b]	2.0–3.0 mg	Formation of hemoglobin; constituent of oxidase enzymes	Anemia; aneurysms; CNS lesions
Fluoride	Seafoods, fluoridated drinking water	1.5–5.0 mg[b]	—	Constituent of tooth enamel; strengthens bones and teeth	Dental decay; osteoporosis

Mineral	Food Sources			Function	Deficiency Symptoms
Iodine	Seafoods, iodized salt	150 mcg	250 mcg	Constituent of thyroxin; regulator of cellular oxidation	Goiter; cretinism
Iron	Organ meats, meats, green leafy vegetables, whole grain breads and cereals.	10 mg (male); 15–18 mg (female)	10 mg (male and post-menopausal female); 20 mg (pre-menopausal female)	Constituent of hemoglobin, myoglobin, catalase, cytochromes, enzyme cofactor	Anemia: fatigue; reduced resistance to colds and infections
Manganese	Organ meats, wheat germ, legumes, nuts	2.5–5.0 mg[b]	—	Cofactor for enzymes; synthesis of mucopoly-saccharides	In animals—sterility, weakness
Molyb-denum	Organ meats, whole grain breads and cereals, legumes, dark green leafy vegetables	75–250 mcg[b]	250 mcg	Constituent of xanthine oxidase, aldehyde oxidase	Stunted growth, reduced food consumption, decreased life expectancy

(continued)

TABLE 16. Essential trace minerals (continued)

Mineral	Best Food Source	RDA (1989)[a]	ODA[b]	Principal Functions	Major Deficiency Symptoms
Selenium	Organ meats, whole grain breads and cereals, vegetables (depending on Se in soil)	70 mcg	200 mcg	Constituent of glutathione peroxidase; inhibits lipid peroxidation	Liver and muscle damage; cardiomyopathy
Zinc	Organ meats, shellfish, wheat germ, legumes	15 mg	15–35 mg	Constituent of insulin and enzymes; regulates taste and growth	Anemia; stunted growth; hypogonadism in male; decreased protein synthesis and wound healing; diminished taste

[a]Recommended Dietary Allowances are established by the Food and Nutrition Board of the National Research Council. The values given are for a normal adult male, 19 to 22 years old.

[b]An estimated range recommended by the Food and Nutrition Board (1989) as safe and adequate daily intakes for healthy people.

[c]Optimal Daily Intake is a theoretical range based on the authors' literature research. If no range is listed, the authors felt there was insufficient evidence to make a recommendation at this time.

Table 17. Tests for iron deficiency and iron-deficiency anemia

Test	Values
Plasma ferritin	Normal: 40–160 mcg/l
	Iron depletion: 20 mcg/l
	Iron-deficiency anemia: <12 mcg/l
Iron binding capacity (TIBC)	Normal: 300–360 mcg/dl
	Iron depletion: 360 mcg/dl
	Iron-deficiency anemia: 410 mcg/dl
Transferrin saturation	Normal: 20%–50%
	Iron depletion: 30%
	Iron-deficiency anemia: <10%
Hemoglobin	Normal: 12–16 g/dl
	Iron-deficiency anemia: <12 g/dl
Hematocrit	Normal: 37%–47%
	Iron-deficiency anemia: <37%

about the authors

Vicki Guercia Caruana is a teacher turned writer who specializes in educational topics for teachers, parents, and children. Vicki seeks to educate and encourage kids and those who live and work with them to strive for excellence. Her best-selling book *Apples & Chalkdust* has sold more than 600,000 copies. She has written more than 80 articles and 20 books and is a frequent guest on national radio and television programs. Vicki speaks at educational, parenting, homeschooling, and writers' conferences. She is also an educational spokesperson whose most recent client is Nintendo. She is also often invited to speak at schools and universities. She has written curriculum for school districts and homeschoolers and desires to provide a quality education for all children. Vicki wants to encourage teachers and teach the rest of American society how to do the same. Her website www.vickicaruana .blogspot.com is devoted to this mission. Vicki lives with her husband and two children in Seminole, Florida.

Kelly Guercia Hammer is a nutritionist and personal trainer. She has a degree in nutrition and fitness from Florida State University and has subsequently trained and been consultant to more than 1,000 individuals. Since 1991, she has worked with corporate executives, athletes, stay-at-home moms, and beginning weight trainers. She worked as a personal health consultant/trainer in New York City at the Waldorf Astoria. Her client list included former mayor Ed Koch at the time. As an independent consultant, Kelly offers workshops on the importance of posture, back health, and balanced lifestyles at spas/resorts and community organizations. Through her business, Hammer Nutritional, Kelly works toward "Building Balance in Families: Mind, Body and Spirit." She lives with her husband and two children in Sylva, North Carolina.